Somebody's Knocking at Your Door
AIDS and the
African-American Church

THE HAWORTH PASTORAL PRESS
Religion and Mental Health
Harold G. Koenig, MD
Senior Editor

New, Recent, and Forthcoming Titles:

A Gospel for the Mature Years: Finding Fulfillment by Knowing and Using Your Gifts by Harold Koenig, Tracy Lamar, and Betty Lamar

Is Religion Good for Your Health? The Effects of Religion on Physical and Mental Health by Harold Koenig

Adventures in Senior Living: Learning How to Make Retirement Meaningful and Enjoyable by J. Lawrence Driskill

Dying, Grieving, Faith, and Family: A Pastoral Care Approach by George W. Bowman

The Pastoral Care of Depression: A Guidebook by Binford W. Gilbert

Understanding Clergy Misconduct in Religious Systems: Scapegoating, Family Secrets, and the Abuse of Power by Candace R. Benyei

What the Dying Teach Us: Lessons on Living by Samuel Lee Oliver

The Pastor's Family: The Challenges of Family Life and Pastoral Responsibilities by Daniel L. Langford

Somebody's Knocking at Your Door: AIDS and the African-American Church by Ronald Jeffrey Weatherford and Carole Boston Weatherford

Grief Education for Caregivers of the Elderly by Junietta Baker McCall

Somebody's Knocking at Your Door
AIDS and the African-American Church

Ronald Jeffrey Weatherford, MDiv
Carole Boston Weatherford, MFA

The Haworth Pastoral Press
An Imprint of The Haworth Press, Inc.
New York • London

Published by

The Haworth Pastoral Press, an imprint of The Haworth Press, Inc., 10 Alice Street, Binghamton, NY 13904-1580

Cover design by Jennifer M. Gaska.

Library of Congress Cataloging-in-Publication Data

Weatherford, Ronald Jeffrey.
    Somebody's knocking at your door : AIDS and the African-American church / Ronald Jeffrey Weatherford, Carole Boston Weatherford.
       p. cm.
    Includes bibliographical references and index.
    ISBN 0-7890-0575-1 (alk. paper).
    1. AIDS (Disease—Religious aspects—Christianity. 2. Afro-American churches. I. Weatherford, Carole Boston, 1956- . II. Title.
BV4460.7.W43 1998
261.8′321969792′008996073—dc21
                                                   98-39344
                                                    CIP

By the time you read
this dedication,
someone else will have been
infected with HIV.

For the living.

R. J. W.
and
C. B. W.

ABOUT THE AUTHORS

Ronald Jeffrey Weatherford, MDiv, is Pastor of the Camp Springs and Garrett's Grove United Methodist Churches in North Carolina and an employee of the United States Postal Service. He has also worked for several other federal agencies, including the National Park Service and the United States Department of Agriculture. Mr. Weatherford is a member of Black Methodists for Church Renewal and the High Point Human Relations Commission. In addition, he serves as an Adjunct Chaplain for the Moses Cone Health Care System.

Carole Boston Weatherford, MFA, MA, is an author and award-winning poet. She has written five children's books, including *My Favorite Toy* and *Juneteenth Jamboree,* and her articles have appeared in *The Christian Science Monitor, Essence, The Washington Post,* and *Charlotte Observer.* Ms. Weatherford's poetry has been published in such journals as *Callaloo, Calyx, African American Review,* and *Slipstream.* In 1995, Ms. Weatherford won the North Carolina Arts Council writer's fellowship and the Furious Flower Poetry Prize, awarded to a promising new poet. In the same year, her poetry volume, *The Tan Chanteuse,* won the North Carolina Writers' Network's Harperprints Chapbook competition. In 1997, Ms. Weatherford won the North Carolina Poetry Society's Caldwell Nixon, Jr. award for her children's poem, *The Griot's Tale.* In addition, she is a member of the North Carolina Writers' Network. When she is not busy writing, Ms. Weatherford conducts performances and residencies at schools and cultural institutions.

CONTENTS

Foreword

When it comes to HIV/AIDS, the African-American community has gone past the crisis stage and is now in a state of emergency. According to the Harvard AIDS Institute, AIDS is now the number one killer of African Americans under the age of fifty-five. While African Americans make up about 12 percent of the American population, they now account for 48 percent of the current AIDS cases in the United States and by the start of the twenty-first century, half of all AIDS cases will be African American. By the year 2005, that number will rise to 60 percent unless we do something about it.

The clarion call issued by Ronald and Carole Weatherford in this book is the call for the African-American church to do something to stop the rapid spread of HIV/AIDS in its community.

The fact of the matter is that HIV/AIDS is entirely preventable. No one has to be infected from this day forward. Unlike airborne diseases, current research indicates that HIV/AIDS is not extremely contagious. Rather it is only acquired through contact with infected body fluids, primarily through unprotected sex or through the sharing of needles in drug usage. So if we stop unprotected sex and the use of dirty needles, we do not need to have even one more additional case of HIV/AIDS in the African-American community. Unfortunately, that is easier said than done.

Although the African-American church has two centuries of history of confronting social justice issues, the church has found it difficult to tackle this issue, which forces us to deal with delicate issues of sexuality (both heterosexuality and homosexuality) and with the high usage of drugs in our community. Yet

Scripture calls us to deal with those who are outcast, those who are ill, and those who are imprisoned. Jesus warned, ". . . just as you did not do it to one of the least of these, you did not do it to me" (Matthew 25:45, NRSV). Indeed, what better place than the church to provide the individual and collective healing of our community!

The media today has convinced most Americans that HIV/ AIDS is a disease of the past and that while it is not curable, it certainly is under control. But, some half a million African Americans are already infected with HIV. Many of these are unable to afford the high cost of the new drugs (upward of $15,000 per year) and others do not live lifestyles that allow them to take these drugs in the highly regimented daily routine in which they must be taken.

Without direct intervention by our community's most significant and trusted social service provider, the black church, hundreds of thousands of others will be infected. The "faces of AIDS" are changing, with more women being infected. By the year 2000 an African-American woman will be nearly twenty times more likely to have AIDS. African-American children are already infected with HIV more than children of all other races combined. African-American teenagers are particularly vulnerable and growing numbers of African-American seniors are being diagnosed with the disease.

Indeed, every day nearly 100 people of color in the United States find out they have AIDS. Only a comprehensive education and prevention program can change these numbers and this book challenges those of us in the church to do more to stop this epidemic.

Finally, the Weatherfords give us examples of churches already deeply involved in ministering to people with HIV/AIDS and who are doing the kind of education and prevention that must be done if a dent is to be made in those projections. These churches call us all to Christ's servant ministry, both to those living with HIV/AIDS and to their families and caretakers. They show us that every black church, no matter where it is located, no matter its size, no matter its resources, can be doing some kind of AIDS ministry.

The fact is that almost everyone in the African-American community now knows someone who is living with, or who has died from this disease. Perhaps it is a family member, a friend, or the child of a friend. AIDS now has a face in just about every black family in America.

Because of those faces we can no longer be silent. Because of the pain of family members who have suffered silently in our churches, unable to share their stories, we can no longer be quiet. Because of the mandate of our Lord and Savior Jesus Christ we must answer the door to those who stand outside knocking.

Bernice Powell Jackson
Executive Director
United Church of Christ
Commission for Racial Justice

Preface

Then Jesus went about all the cities and villages, teaching in their synagogues, and proclaiming the good news of the Kingdom, and curing every disease and every sickness. When he saw the crowds, he had compassion for them, because they were harassed and helpless, like sheep without a shepherd.

Matthew 9:35-36

In 1982, my wife and co-author, Carole, read a *New York* magazine article titled "The Gay Plague." She photocopied the piece and sent it to a gay friend in New York along with a note warning, "Please be careful." By the disease's second decade, her friend's younger brother, also homosexual, had become infected. When Carole read that article, she had no idea that heterosexuals were also at risk.

In 1985, while a student minister in Greensboro, North Carolina, I preached my first AIDS sermon. I was surprised that the sermon, which advocated condom use, was so well received among the church's older adults.

It was through my primary job as a letter carrier, however, that I first encountered the ravages of AIDS. Loitering, drugs, and prostitution plagued the low- to moderate-income African-American neighborhood I served. On my mail route, I noticed several young men who appeared to be getting sicker and sicker. Instead of hanging on corners, they sat on their mothers' porches in bathrobes. When I inquired about their health the men replied that they had "the disease." One by one, they died.

Several years later, I learned that some of my friends and family members were infected. All have since died.

This book grew out of my master's thesis at Shaw Divinity School in Raleigh, North Carolina. The thesis examined the African-American church's response to AIDS. My research uncovered several scattered African-American AIDS ministries, but found that most African-American congregations had not responded to the growing epidemic.

This book builds on my thesis research with surveys of African-American AIDS ministries and interviews of leading AIDS advocates representing religious and nonprofit groups. With help from Sharon H. Lipscomb, director of client services at High Point (North Carolina's Triad Health Project), I also conducted focus groups involving African-Americans living with AIDS. The participants—whose names have been changed in this book—spoke candidly about the lifestyle implications and spiritual impact of AIDS. This book also examines reasons behind the church's apathy as well as rationales for action. We also discuss Africa, where AIDS is taking its greatest toll.

I encourage both clergy and laity to use this book to open dialogue about AIDS and develop compassionate ministries for people in our communities and around the world who are infected with and affected by the disease.

Ronald J. Weatherford

Chapter 1

Why the African-American Church?

Long before the civil rights movement. . . we went to the
church for everything. The church was our social service
organization as well as our spiritual service organization.
The church is still being looked on . . . by large segments of
our community as being central in our lives.[1]

Jim Harvey
Executive Director
New City Health Center
Chicago, Illinois
(quoted in *Positively Aware,* 1997)

In the nation's predominately African-American inner cities,
urban ills—drugs, crime, and poverty—are literally knocking at
the doors of some churches. Now, some African-American leaders are urging the church to join the fight against AIDS. Doesn't
the African-American church have enough to do?

With collective and individual power far surpassing any single
civil rights organization, the African-American church is a sleep-
ing giant. In the 1990 book, *The Black Church in the African-*
American Experience, C. Eric Lincoln and Lawrence H. Mamiya
estimated that 23.7 million African Americans are church members. A 1997 Gallup Poll found that weekly church attendance is
much higher among African Americans than among whites:

40 percent versus 29 percent. Emmett D. Carson, author of *A Hand Up: Black Philanthropy and Self-Help in America*, reports that 90 percent of an African American's charitable contributions go to the church and other religious organizations—giving what Lincoln and Mamiya say approaches roughly $2 billion annually.[2]

In addition, the African-American community is undergoing a spiritual renaissance. This trend is evident in the growth of African-American megachurches, the popularity of spiritual self-help books, and the growing interest in spiritual retreats and discussion groups. At the same time, African-American baby boomers are returning to church, seeking inspiration, fellowship, and constructive ways to revitalize their communities.

Given these trends, the nation's 65,000 African-American churches would appear to have reason to rejoice. A ten-year study by Lincoln and Mamiya, however, found that African-American clergy perceive several problems, including: lack of evangelism, secularization, sin, inadequate finances, criticism of leadership, and aging memberships. While 80 percent of African Americans went to church two decades ago, only 40 percent attend today. Amidst these mounting challenges, the African-American church's delayed response to AIDS is somewhat understandable.

POWER IN THE PEWS

Perennial problems aside, the African-American church is uniquely suited to address AIDS in the African-American community. Since slavery times, the African-American church has taken the lead in the African-American community. In fact, the first national African-American leader—Bishop Richard Allen—hailed from the African Methodist Episcopal Church.

African-American churches were the first communally built institutions in some Reconstruction-era communities. The churches, in turn, established hundreds of schools and colleges without government funding. In many areas, these church-run schools were the only educational institutions open to African Americans. Churches continue to support more private African-American colleges and universities than any other institution.

The founding of educational institutions is by far the church's most lasting, but by no means its only, contribution. Early on, African-American churches promoted economic uplift. By 1900, the African-American church served as the community's social hub, as a funding source and recruitment arm for organizations such as the NAACP and the National Urban League, and as an incubator for publications, hospitals, and financial institutions. Some African-American banks and insurance companies actually began as burial societies, mutual aid societies, and benevolent associations in African-American churches and fraternal orders.

This focus on self-help continues today. In low-income African-American communities, the church is the one enduring institution that can secure major credit for community development. African-American churches operate more day care centers, construct more affordable income housing, and administer more tutorial programs than all others institutions in the black community combined.[3]

Since the days when northern African-American churches were stations along the Underground Railroad, liberation theology has permeated the African-American church's preaching and teachings, and African-American clergy have helped wage the freedom struggle. A roll call of the twentieth century's leading activists would certainly include these clergymen: Harlem Congressman Adam Clayton Powell; James Farmer, cofounder of the Congress of Racial Equality; Vernon Johns, Martin Luther King Jr.'s predecessor at Montgomery, Alabama's Dexter Avenue Baptist Church; Leon Sullivan, founder of Opportunities Industrialization Centers of America; former Southern Christian Leadership Conference President Joseph Lowery; former NAACP Executive Director Benjamin Hooks; former United Nations Ambassador and Atlanta

Mayor Andrew Young; Rainbow/PUSH Coalition President Jesse Jackson; and, of course, Martin Luther King Jr. and Malcolm X.

It is no coincidence that the African-American church has also been a breeding ground for politicians. From Reconstruction-era Congressman Hiram Revels to New York Congressman Floyd Flake, the pulpit has catapulted African-American preachers into seats of power. If there was previously any doubt, Jesse Jackson's 1984 and 1988 presidential campaigns proved once and for all that African-American churches could get out the vote. Equally important is the role of the African-American church in grooming community leaders.

The church is the oldest institution that African Americans can truly call their own. The African-American church is a city of refuge and source of empowerment for African Americans. They invest not only considerable time and money in the church, but also their hope. That could explain why African-American churches are prime targets of white supremacist hate groups.

Racists, however, are not the only ones who recognize the power of the African-American church. So do major marketers. Segmented Marketing Services, Inc., an African-American-owned firm in Winston-Salem, North Carolina, developed the SMSI Church Family Network, a promotion system that distributes product samples to urban African-American churchgoers. With the capacity to reach half of the nation's African-American households, the Church Family Network taps into the grapevine, a vital communications link in the black community. Studies of African-American consumer behavior show that word-of-mouth advertising wields more influence when the endorsement comes from perceived peer group leaders such as pastors.

POWER OF THE PULPIT

For generations, the church was the sole arbiter of social norms in the African-American community. Though the power of the pulpit waned slightly as church attendance declined, what African-American preachers say is still often regarded by many churchgoers as gospel. And once parishioners leave the sanctuary, they spread the message throughout the community.

In a February 1998 interview, AIDS advocate Pernessa Seele, founder and director of The Balm in Gilead, said, "The black pulpit's reach goes far beyond the doors of the church."[4]

With faithful followers in the pews and a constituency in the community, the African-American church has the clout to disseminate mass information and mobilize volunteers. That's just what's needed to address the AIDS crisis.

The church "could do a lot in terms of mass information," activist minister Al Sharpton said in a February 1998 interview. "It can give a platform to people who can mass educate and mass inform. It can use its political power to influence those in public office about AIDS policy and funding.

"Once the African-American church makes up its mind," Sharpton continued, "there are no obstacles that can stop it. It has not been challenged. The biggest obstacle is its will."[5]

If faith indeed moves mountains, African-American churches must summon that faith to tackle the AIDS epidemic. "If we're going to address the AIDS issue effectively," said Pernessa Seele, "we must engage the black church."[6]

Public policies on welfare, drug abuse, law enforcement, health care, education, and affirmative action have led some African-American leaders to believe that the government considers minorities and the poor to be expendable. If that is the case, the African-American community should probably not rely on the government to stem the spread of AIDS.

Unlike other problems the African-American church has addressed, AIDS is not merely a quality-of-life issue, it is also a life-or-death issue. On AIDS Awareness Sunday in 1995, Reverend Jeremiah Wright of Chicago's Trinity United Church of Christ asked parishioners to stand if they have had a friend or family member die of AIDS. One-third of the 2,000-member congregation stood up. This is a state of emergency. But this is by no means the first time that the African-American community has endured suffering.

NOBODY KNOWS THE TROUBLE I'VE SEEN

"The African-American church," said George McKinney, pastor of Saint Stephen's Church of God in Christ in Los Angeles, can "deal with the urban crisis, because we have been in the crucible of pain."[7]

Indeed, the American legacy of racism is so agonizing that tennis champion and humanitarian Arthur Ashe declared in his posthumous memoir *Days of Grace:* "Race is for me a more onerous burden than AIDS."[8] Neither wealth nor celebrity made him immune to bigotry or to HIV. Ashe, who contracted AIDS from a blood transfusion following 1988 heart surgery, died in 1993.

In African-American communities across the country, AIDS continues to inflict pain and claim lives. Just as the church collects benevolence offerings for needy families and conducts health screenings for senior citizens, it must also bring its influence and energy to bear in the fight against AIDS. The epidemic presents an opportunity to not only save lives, but to redefine the church for the twenty-first century.

The African-American church has long understood the holistic nature of the gospel. To minister to the whole person and the whole community, many churches have ventured into the business, social, and political arenas, developing businesses and real estate, creating jobs, mobilizing voters, and tackling problems such as substance abuse, crime, teen pregnancy, and AIDS. The African-American church, however, needs to expand its scope even more.

Churches and community-based organizations need to find ways to partner in the delivery of AIDS services and prevention education. This synergy is crucial as AIDS advances in the African-American community.

In July 1997, Mario Cooper, a trustee of the International Association of Physicians in AIDS Care, briefed the Congressional Black Caucus on the AIDS crisis. "African-American leaders," he lamented, "have virtually ignored HIV/AIDS. We must throw aside the shackles of ignorance, homophobia, and fear, and grasp this window of opportunity to help our communities."[9]

Cooper led the Harvard AIDS Institute's October 1996 Leading for Life Summit. At the event—billed as an emergency summit—members of the Harvard AIDS Institute blasted the African-American church and prominent civil rights organizations for sitting on the sidelines as AIDS took its toll on their congregations and communities.

During the Harvard summit, Henry Louis Gates, chair of the university's W.E.B. DuBois Institute, called the disease "our generation's war."[10] Regardless of whether Christian soldiers join the fight, AIDS is ravaging the African-American community. Ultimately, truth will be the most effective weapon in this battle. And the church is the most revered messenger of truth. The African-American church has a responsibility to lends its voice and leverage its strength to help combat AIDS.

The church must first help the community to overcome homophobia and fears stemming from misconceptions about AIDS transmission by opening dialogue on sexuality. The 1997 National Black Religious Summit on Sexuality, sponsored by the Religious Coalition for Reproductive Choice, encouraged such discussions. Setting the tone for the Summit, Reverend Carlton Veazey stressed, "To help our brothers and sisters live the abundant life, our ministry must be holistic in its approach, addressing the sexual aspect of each person. We must talk about areas of sexuality which have traditionally been unspoken in the church, including. . . HIV/AIDS."[11]

Today, thriving African-American churches—including mega-churches with huge congregations and budgets to match—appear to have one thing in common. They work all week long to uplift the community. Instead of simply looking up to God, they look down to help the disenfranchised and relieve suffering. Apparently, the spirit of caring is contagious, for members flock to churches that face crises head on.

"Whatever the church stands for, it must stand for ministering to the least of these," Veazey asserted during an interview.[12]

A health and social problem, AIDS is one of the most serious threats facing descendants of Africa since the slave trade. The African-American church is slowly awakening to the enormity of the crisis. During the disease's first decade, the majority of African-American churches ignored the disease's impact rather than grapple with the thorny issues surrounding AIDS transmission. Because HIV/AIDS was stigmatized as a gay plague, mainstream churches initially adopted a condescending attitude toward the disease and those infected with it. Such attitudes softened over time as the public came to understand that HIV infects people without regard to race, ethnicity, class, age, gender, or sexual orientation.

Where the African-American church now stands on HIV/AIDS is difficult to pinpoint. Some religious bodies still consider the virus God's wrath for carnal sins. Other denominations have appealed to their followers to be compassionate to those living with AIDS. And some autonomous African-American churches have not ventured into that territory. Suffice it to say, the collective African-American church has no homogeneous position on HIV/AIDS. Many African-American churches have steered clear of both AIDS and homosexuality, though both issues confront the African-American community. Their silence speaks volumes.

In February 1997, a coalition of African-American ministers in Boston held a press conference to apologize for their lack of leadership in mobilizing the church against AIDS. They urged local churches to join the battle against AIDS. In addition, they also acknowledged that clergy must provide moral and spiritual leadership if African-American communities are to survive this epidemic and remain emotionally intact.[13]

AIDS is striking down more and more African Americans in their prime. And AIDS is on the rise among older adults—the age group most likely to attend church. If the epidemic continues unchecked, there will eventually be few faithful to fill African-American church pews. For the African-American church, then, getting involved in the AIDS issue is a matter of survival.

Progressive churches recognize AIDS as an opportunity to be an embracing community, to save not only souls, but lives as well. In meeting the need for compassion and caring, however, the church must be cautious not to abandon its prophetic role in society. In responding to the need for intervention on the AIDS issue, the church need not abdicate its concern or relax its standards about lifestyle and behavior choices, especially since poor choices often result in people becoming less than what God intended for them.

The biblical record clearly states that man's identity is reconciled to God. God accepts human frailties. As such, the church, acting as the visible body of Christ, has an obligation to help and comfort those in need.

As the African-American spiritual, "'Tis the Old Ship of Zion," attests, the church has traditionally answered that call:

Tis the old ship of Zion, 'tis the old ship of Zion
'tis the old ship of Zion, get on board, get on board.
It has landed many a thousand, it has landed many a thousand,
it has landed many a thousand, get on board, get on board.

In his 1974 book, *The Black Experience in Religion*, theologian C. Eric Lincoln noted, "Beyond its purely religious function, as critical as that is, the Afro-American church has in its historical role been the champion of our freedom and the hallmark of our civilization" (p. 55).[14]

The African-American church has helped millions navigate the stormy sea of prejudice. It has lifted boats at the bottom, been a beacon for lost souls, and a lifeline for drowning spirits. The AIDS epidemic warrants similar leadership.

Let this be an invitation for the church to get on board.

Chapter 2

Two in Five: AIDS Statistics
in the African-American Community

How many of us will be infected before it becomes our problem? How many will develop AIDS? How many will die? Three hundred thousand cases later, I still wonder. . .[1]

Phill Wilson
AIDS policy expert

NAMING A NEW PLAGUE

In February 1998, David Ho, MD, of the Aaron Diamond AIDS Research Center announced that the earliest known case of human immunodeficiency virus (HIV) and acquired immunodeficiency syndrome (AIDS) infection had been identified in an African blood sample collected in 1959 from a man living in Kinshasa, Democratic Republic of Congo (now Zaire). Researchers speculate that HIV/AIDS may have first infected green monkeys and then crossed over to the human population. The virus has mutated several times over the years.

The first HIV/AIDS cases were diagnosed in 1981. In the late 1970s, rare types of cancer and infections were reported to be increasing among previously healthy persons. Physicians observed that these opportunistic illnesses rarely struck those with normal, healthy immune systems. This medical trend was first documented in homosexual and bisexual men. Soon, however, the disease was observed in intravenous (IV) drug users, hemophiliacs, and recipients of blood transfusions. Sexual partners of infected persons were also contracting the disease. Medical researchers eventually determined that the disease spread in three ways: (1) through sexual intercourse (vaginal or anal) or oral sex with an HIV-positive partner; (2) by having the blood of an infected person enter the body, a situation most likely among intravenous drug users who share needles;[2] and (3) by HIV-positive mothers to unborn children either in the womb or during childbirth.

Those who have tested positive for HIV, but do not exhibit the full blown symptoms of AIDS, are referred to as HIV positive. The U.S. Centers for Disease Control and Prevention (CDC) estimates that 900,000 people in the United States have been infected with HIV.[3] And people who are HIV-positive can potentially infect others with the disease. By June 1997, the CDC had counted 612,078 AIDS cases and 379,528 AIDS-related deaths in the United States.

AIDS DOESN'T DISCRIMINATE

Although African Americans make up only 13 percent of the total U.S. population, they account for 35 percent of AIDS cases reported to the CDC. As of December 1996, 120,000 African Americans had died from AIDS. As many as 500,000 African Americans could be infected with HIV.

In 1996, for the first time, African Americans represented a larger proportion (41 percent) of newly reported AIDS cases than whites (38 percent). African Americans are more than six times as likely as whites to be infected with HIV/AIDS. AIDS is the leading killer of African Americans under age fifty-five, before heart disease, cancer, and homicide. Over one in five reported HIV infections occurred in African Americans under age thirty.

And AIDS kills twice as many African-American men aged twenty-five to forty-four as homicide.

Racial and ethnic disparities in AIDS incidence, however, are more striking among women and children. AIDS is the leading cause of death for African-American women aged twenty-five to forty-four. Of all AIDS cases in women reported to the CDC in 1996, two out of three were among African-American women. As of June 1997, more than twice as many African-American women had been infected as white women. AIDS contracted through IV drug use is seventeen times more common among African-American women than whites. Of babies born with AIDS, six out of ten are African American. Most troubling, more African-American children are infected with HIV than children of all other races and ethnicities combined.

AIDS also affects children in a way that is often overlooked. The disease has orphaned nearly 60,000 children under the age of eighteen. If current rates continue, the CDC estimates that by the year 2000 there could be as many as 125,000 AIDS orphans in the United States.

HIV/AIDS RISK FACTORS AND TRANSMISSION MODES

Major modes of AIDS transmission also vary widely among racial and ethnic groups. White men, for example, are more than twice as likely as African Americans to contract AIDS through homosexual contact. African-American men are more than twice as likely as white men to contract AIDS through IV drug use or heterosexual contact. In addition, a study of 65,000 HIV-positive men published in the *American Journal of Public Health* found that African-American men are twice as likely as white men to be bisexual, a factor that increases the AIDS risk among African-American women.[4]

HIV/AIDS affects and infects a broad cross-section of people in the United States regardless of age, race, gender, or sexual orientation. CDC statistics show that large metropolitan areas have the largest concentrations of AIDS cases, but the disease is present in all U.S. populations. Overall, however, the African-American community is at higher risk of HIV infection. Though race and ethnicity in and of themselves are not risk factors, race is a marker for other factors—such as geographic location and poverty—that compound risk. African Americans, for example, are more likely to live in inner cities, a foci of the epidemic.

In a 1995 *FDA Consumer* magazine article, Paul Denning, an epidemiologist in the CDC's AIDS Surveillance Branch, explained,

> Because the virus is very prevalent in these communities, the chances or odds that a person's sexual partner may be infected with HIV are increased. One must also consider that injection drug use and other substance abuse, which are concentrated in urban areas, have played a major role in the spread of AIDS. (p. 3)[5]

In addition, inner city residents are more likely to be unemployed, poor, and illiterate—conditions that correlate with limited access to health education, preventive services, and medical care. It follows that African-Americans who live in inner cities are less likely to seek treatment and undergo tests for medical problems and to know their HIV status. These factors raise the risk for disease.

AIDS' initial stigma as a gay plague led some African-American families to keep their AIDS-infected relatives in seclusion. This secrecy not only perpetuated the myth that the disease only affected homosexuals, but bred denial. Consequently, many at risk failed to practice preventive measures, such as abstinence and condom use.

The rate of incarceration among African-American males also increases the AIDS risk in the African-American community. An estimated one million African-American men are incarcerated.[6] Through unprotected anal sex, a common practice among inmates, the virus spreads throughout prison populations. Blind testing in several big city prisons suggests that as many one in four inmates could be HIV positive. Upon their release from prison, the inmates—often unaware of their HIV status—unknowingly spread the infection to female sex partners.

HIV/AIDS RATES RISING
AMONG AFRICAN AMERICANS

Many Americans falsely believe that homosexuals and IV drug users are the major populations at risk for HIV/AIDS. Since AIDS was first identified among gay men the demographics of the disease have changed drastically. When the HIV/AIDS mode of transmission was understood to involve sexual behavior, the gay community took action to limit the spread of the disease. Gay organizations promoted safe sex practices and advocated open communication about sexual issues. These efforts resulted in a gradual decrease of HIV infection among the gay population.

In 1996, AIDS cases declined in all racial or ethnic groups, except African Americans, for whom the rate of incidence was unchanged, perhaps due to lack of health care insurance to cover the $14,000-per-year prescription cost of promising new treatments that delay the onset of AIDS symptoms. In a survey of 700 HIV-infected New Yorkers, researchers from the Columbia University School of Public Health found that only 12 percent of African-American patients were taking protease inhibitors, compared to 33 percent of white patients.

Despite a nationwide drop in reports of new AIDS cases, the incidence of new AIDS diagnosis among heterosexuals continued to rise. In fact, the greatest proportionate increases occurred among African Americans and Hispanics infected heterosexually.

AIDS is also on the rise among older Americans, who, contrary to popular belief, are still sexually active. The most prevalent risks for older adults are multiple sexual partners or having a partner with behavioral risk. Most older people believe they are not at risk if they are heterosexual and do not inject drugs. Since they are not worried about pregnancy, older people are less likely to use condoms. Further, the elderly lack sufficient education about the transmission and spread of the disease.

In an interview, Reverend Charles Matthews, coordinator of Baltimore-based Churches United Against AIDS, reported knowing an octogenarian church deacon who contracted HIV/AIDS from one of the young prostitutes who frequented a senior citizens' apartment building when monthly retirement checks arrived. As a deacon, he not only visited the church's sick and shut-ins, but widows as well. He passed the virus along to a widow with whom he was intimate.

During a July 1997 health forum hosted by Congressman Louis Stokes (D-OH), Abdul Alim Muhammed, MD, minister of health and human services for the Nation of Islam, indicated that 30 percent of the student body at a Southeast Washington, DC, high school tested positive for HIV. Nationwide, African Americans account for more than one in three AIDS cases among teenage males. Similarly, more than twice as many African-American teenage girls have AIDS as their white and Hispanic counterparts.

The CDC has spotted some troubling trends among youth. Many American teenagers are engaging in behaviors that may put them at risk of acquiring HIV infection, other sexually transmitted diseases, or infections associated with drug injection. Recent CDC studies conducted every two years in high schools (grades 9 to 12) consistently indicate that by the twelfth grade, approximately three-fourths of high school students have had sexual intercourse; less than half report consistent use of latex condoms; and about one-fifth have had more than four sex partners. Many students report using alcohol or drugs when they have sex and, in the most recent survey, one in sixty-two high school students reported having injected an illegal drug.

According to the Harvard AIDS Institute, if current HIV infection and AIDS-incidence rates continue, by the year 2005, 60 percent of all AIDS cases in the United States could be among African Americans.[7]

Otis Tillman, MD, a family practitioner in High Point, North Carolina, has treated many AIDS patients. In his inspirational book, *A Prescription for the Soul: Prayers & Meditations*, he shared an anecdote about a young patient crushed by an HIV-positive diagnosis. "This scenario has been replayed many times over the past ten years with different patients," the physician wrote, "but the outcome remains the same—broken dreams and wasted lives."[8]

Tillman offered this prayer for people living with AIDS:

Dear Lord,
When the uncertainties of life cause us to question the very foundation of our spiritual existence, we turn with faithful hearts to You. Crises of this nature cause us to realize how dependent we are on Your spirit to support our lives. May we forever be sustained by Your grace and guided by the light of Your love. Amen.[9] (p. 13)

Chapter 3

Sex—A Hang-Up
in the African-American Church

They [black preachers] speak about sex in any form as if it's cancer. We need the church to help us deal with the prejudice and the bias that we face as we're trying to fight this epidemic.[1]

David Satcher, MD
U.S. Surgeon General

"More devastating than the physical disease known as AIDS is the spiritual disease (Acquired Iniquity Devilish Sins). And the only way to kill its virus is to take daily dosages of the Word of God," declared Robert Thomas, a Nashville newspaper columnist known as "The Road Scholar."[2]

This simplistic analogy implies that those infected with HIV/AIDS are victims of their own spiritual failings. Such views, which proliferate among African-American clergy, provide justification for some churches to withhold compassion from people living with AIDS.

During the first decade of AIDS, some African-American ministers refused to preside over funerals of AIDS victims, and funeral directors refused to bury them. Most African-American clergy are more tolerant nowadays, though some pastors' funeral homilies still diminish AIDS victims' spiritual worth.

Despite the toll AIDS is taking on the African-American community, homosexuality has rarely been openly discussed in the

African-American church. This does not mean that homosexuality was not condemned from the pulpit. On the contrary, outspoken anti-gay preachers do not hesitate to use the pulpit to condemn gay lifestyles. These pastors' homophobic stances hinder, rather than foster, the African-American church's ability to address the growing AIDS epidemic in the African-American community.

To respond to the suffering caused by AIDS, the African-American church must work to overcome its own polarizing beliefs regarding the disease and homosexuality.

IN PURSUIT OF PURITY

Sexual purity is a dominant theme in Biblical treatments of sexual morality. In the ancient sense, purity required individuals to avoid actions that would defile them. From the ancients' perspective, everything that individuals touched could render them dirty. Modern society does not have purity rules in the strict sense of the Mosaic Codes. However, we know from experience that we instinctively try to rid our lives of dirt.

The codes for purity contained in the Torah were based on the conviction that God was holy and that God's chosen people were to also be holy. The Torah delineates the holy and unholy. The priests were the most clean and the lepers were the outcasts. This was the world into which Jesus was born. He bridged the chasm between those who pointed fingers and those who needed help. He did not shun the unclean, but rather sought to heal through His touch. His actions demonstrated inclusiveness. From the standpoint of Christ's actions, holiness means that those who suffer are welcome and belong at the table.

In the modern world, society's lepers are not physically isolated as they were under Mosaic Law. People living with AIDS (PLWAs), however, often suffer isolation once they disclose their illness. Government-sponsored public awareness campaigns have highlighted the fact that AIDS is not transmitted through casual contact. But because AIDS infection usually amounts to a death sentence, many otherwise rational people fear contact with those infected. When public awareness of the viral infection peaked, many suggested some sort of quarantine for those infected with the disease. AIDS activists, however, charged that a quarantine would be discriminatory.

Though AIDS discrimination is a recent phenomenon, discrimination against homosexuals has been around for a long time. Throughout history, the Bible has been used to discriminate against homosexuals.

BIBLE UNCLEAR ON HOMOSEXUALITY

The African-American church sweeps eroticism under the rug, but most congregations don't even give homosexuality a foot in the door. Fundamentalists of both stripes—African American and white—fall back on Biblical references to condemn homosexuality. Opponents of gay rights often cite Genesis 19:1-25, claiming that God destroyed the city of Sodom because of homosexuality. A critical look at these verses refutes this claim. In the story, two angels are sent by God to the city. Lot invites the travelers to stay in his home. Ancient travelers, in the days before hotels and motels, depended on the kindness of strangers. Hospitality codes required hosts to offer food, shelter, and protection to travelers.

While preparing for bed, the people of Sodom converge on Lot's house demanding that the angels come out so that they might know them. To protect the angels, Lot offers his two virgin daughters instead. This suggests that Lot knew his neighbors were heterosexual. The mob refuses and the angels pull Lot back inside and render the crowd blind. The angels warn Lot to gather his family and leave the city before God destroys it.

Confusion over this passage has to do with the phrase to
"know them." The Hebrew word "yadha," which translates as "to
know," has various meanings throughout the Bible. The most
common meaning is to "have thorough knowledge of." In some
cases, "yadha" may have meant to have sex with. In this case, it
was clear that the townspeople wanted to have sex with the
angels. The point that many readers miss is that the people
wanted to commit an act of violence against the angels. In Ezekiel 16:48-50, the reason for Sodom's destruction is made clear.
According to Ezekiel, the sins of Sodom were pride, laziness,
greed, idolatry, being inhospitable, and neglecting the needs of
the poor. There is no mention of homosexuality in either Ezekiel
or Genesis, nor is homosexuality mentioned elsewhere in scrip-
tural accounts of Sodom.

Two of the most widely used verses to condemn homosexuality come from Leviticus. Leviticus 18:22 states, "You shall not
lie with male as with a woman; it is an abomination." Likewise,
Leviticus 20:13 declares, "If a man lies with a male as with a
woman, both of them have committed an abomination; they shall
be put to death." The word "abomination" in these two verses
means something detestable to God because it is unclean or
unjust. It is usually cited in association with Canaanite religious
practice of cult prostitution.

When treading the Levitical Code, one must keep in mind that
these passages were written as a code and manual for Israelite
priests. It is unfair for modern Christians to cite these passages to
justify denying personhood to those engaged in homosexual lifestyles. After all, many other rules and rituals of the Levitical
Code no longer apply.

Although the Old Testament condemns homosexual and heterosexual cult activity, it does not say that these persons should
be excluded from loving and committed relationships.

JESUS NEVER BASHED GAYS

Opponents of homosexual lifestyles also look to the New Testament epistles of Paul. Romans 1:26, for example, deals with the Laws of Nature: "For this reason God gave them up to degrading passions. Their women exchange natural intercourse for unnatural. . . ." Paul was writing in response to those Christians who had given in to the corruption of paganism and practices that were inconsistent with the truth. These Christians had walked in the knowledge of the faith, but had abandoned the way of God and had given in to self-gratification.

In 1 Corinthians 6:9 and 1 Timothy 1:10, Paul addresses those who are morally weak and deals with the homosexual and heterosexual cult religious practices of his time. These writings attempt to draw nonbelievers to the faith. Because Paul did not directly address the gay lifestyle, we cannot say with certainty that Paul condemned homosexuals.

Further, Jesus himself was silent on the subject. The fact that Jesus said nothing in the Scriptures about homosexuality may indicate that this wasn't one of his chief concerns.

In a February 1998 interview, Pernessa Seele concluded:

> Homosexuality is the scapegoat. Sexuality is the barrier for addressing AIDS in the African-American church. We've never dealt with the issues of sexual abuse or incest. AIDS is bringing the chickens home to roost. We have never dealt with these issues and now we have to.[3]

SOME DENOMINATIONAL VIEWS ON HOMOSEXUALITY AND AIDS

Policies on homosexuality vary widely among mainline and African-American denominations. These positions shed light on the local congregation's attitudes regarding gay lifestyles and their responses to the AIDS epidemic.

Of the historically African-American denominations, only the A.M.E. and A.M.E. Zion Church made public their positions on homosexuality and AIDS. The A.M.E. Church accepts gay members, but does not perform same-sex marriages or ordain homosexual ministers. Similarly, the A.M.E. Zion Church condemns homosexuality but not homosexuals. The denomination does not sanction same-sex marriages or ordain gay ministers. Both denominations call for compassionate responses to AIDS.

Congregations affiliated with the historically black Progressive National Baptist Convention (PNBC), the National Baptist Convention, U.S.A. (NBCUSA), and National Baptist Convention have local autonomy. The NBCUSA's articles of faith, however, state that unrepenting sinners are condemned by God and that Christians are obligated to provide for the sick. In 1996, the NBCUSA called on the World Council of Churches to condemn stereotyping AIDS as a disease of people of color. The PNBC opposes all forms of discrimination and supports universal human liberation.

The PNBC and NBCUSA joined the five other African-American denominations and religious organizations—the National Baptist Convention of America, Church of God in Christ, A.M.E. Church, A.M.E. Zion Church, and C.M.E. Church—in endorsing The Balm in Gilead. An AIDS education and advocacy organization, the New York-based Balm in Gilead represents African-American religious groups on the Council of National Religious AIDS Networks, a body of the AIDS Interfaith Network.

Several mainline denominations with significant African-American memberships have adopted positions on AIDS and homosexuality. The United Methodist Church, Presbyterian Church, U.S.A., Episcopal Church, and Evangelical Lutheran Church in America accept homosexual members, and advocate AIDS ministries. None of these denominations, however, sanction same-sex marriages or ordain gay ministers. In 1997, the

Episcopal Church apologized to gay members and the gay community for years of rejection by the church. The United Methodist and Episcopalian denominations have called for efforts to address racial inequities suffered by minorities living with AIDS.

Among American mainline churches, the United Church of Christ (UCC) is considered the most welcoming to gay and lesbian people as members and ministers. The UCC General Synod has ruled that sexual orientation, in and of itself, not be a barrier to ordination. The ordination policies, however, of the UCC's 204 autonomous associations vary widely. Some oppose, while others affirm, gay clergy. The UCC challenges congregations to minister to PLWAs and combat the spread of the disease.

In comparison to the UCC's policies, the stances of the Roman Catholic Church, Southern Baptists, and Pentecostals are more conservative. The Catholic Church advocates AIDS ministries but promotes abstinence rather than condom use. It accepts homosexual members, but opposes gay rights, and bans same-sex marriages and the ordination of practicing homosexuals. The Southern Baptist Convention opposes promoting safe sex and has repeatedly spoken out against gay rights. The United Pentecostal Church International opposes gay rights, referring to homosexuality as a "satanic snare."

AFRICAN AMERICANS' ATTITUDES ABOUT AIDS

Research shows that AIDS stigma among African Americans was predicted principally by attitudes toward gay men and by beliefs about casual contact. African Americans are about 50 percent more likely than whites to know or have known a person with AIDS or HIV. Of 607 African Americans surveyed from September 1990 to February 1991, more than 85 percent indicated that personal contact with people living with HIV/AIDS had significantly influenced their attitudes. African Americans who had such contact were less likely to blame or avoid people living with HIV/AIDS. Similarly, data suggested that individuals who know someone with HIV/AIDS were more willing to interact with PLWAs than were individuals who had no prior personal contact with PLWAs. More than 35 percent of the African-American respondents were very or somewhat afraid of people infected with HIV/AIDS.[4]

The nationwide study conducted by the Survey Research Center at the University of California at Berkeley found that AIDS-related stigmas are manifested in both the African-American and white communities. More than 35 percent of African Americans were very or somewhat afraid of people infected with HIV/AIDS. The research also pointed to common misconceptions about the transmission of HIV/AIDS. More than half of African-American respondents thought that the virus could potentially be transmitted through a drinking glass, cough, sneeze, or insect bite. Nearly half thought the virus could be transmitted through public toilets. And nearly one in four thought it could be transmitted through kissing on the cheek.[5]

In November 1991 basketball star Earvin "Magic" Johnson's public disclosure of his HIV-positive status brought AIDS out of the shadows and drove home the message that AIDS was not just a disease of homosexuals and heroin users. His shocking announcement had the greatest influence on the attitudes of low-income African Americans.[6] In the wake of his announcement, Gleghorn, Kilbourn, and Celentano found that the number of African-American sexually transmitted-disease patients who vowed to use condoms more than tripled.[7] Kalichman, Russell, Hunter, and Sarwer speculated that Johnson's revelation might soften African-American men's attitudes toward PLWAs in much the same way as a personal relationship with someone infected with HIV.[8]

Since the disease was first identified, HIV/AIDS has been socially defined by stigmas already attached to the marginalized groups that the CDC designated as at high risk for HIV infection: homosexuals, heroin users, and Haitian immigrants. Consequently, public reactions to AIDS reflected prejudices against homosexuals, drug users, people of color, and immigrants.

In his 1996 book *One More River to Cross*, African-American gay social commentator Keith Boykin contrasted the outpouring of emotion for juvenile AIDS victims and the sympathy for heterosexual AIDS victims with the cold shoulder given gay AIDS victims. He wrote, "The black community, like other communities, has developed some compassion toward children, heterosexuals, and celebrities infected with the virus. But the concern often evaporates when the victims are homosexuals" (pp. 121-122).[9]

A 1997 Gallup Poll of the general population showed that Americans are less concerned than they were in 1987 about contracting HIV/AIDS and they also know more about the disease's transmission. The respondents were also less critical and afraid of those who get AIDS. In 1987, 43 percent felt AIDS was a punishment for moral decline. Only 31 percent believed that by 1997. Forty-three percent of those responding to the 1987 survey said they avoided associating with people who might have AIDS. By 1997, only 15 percent indicated taking such precautions. Nevertheless, just under half of the 872 respondents think people with HIV/AIDS should be required to carry a card indicating they are infected.[10]

A 1988 General Social Survey funded by the National Science Foundation revealed that people respond to AIDS based on their view of God.[11] The research also showed that members of traditional denominations, such as Southern Baptists and Roman Catholics, are more conservative in their approach to AIDS. Notably, these denominations also oppose teaching safe sex to prevent AIDS transmission.

A 1997 report on a nationwide Kaiser Family Foundation survey revealed that 35 percent of the 1,200 respondents knew someone who had or died from HIV/AIDS, compared to 2 percent in 1983 and 39 percent in 1995. Among the parents surveyed, 52 percent were very concerned that their child(ren) might become infected.[12]

Although these attitudinal trends are encouraging, the African-American church can take little credit for the enlightenment and compassion that has led to greater acceptance. A study of African-American ministers in New York City, for example, revealed that some hesitated to address the AIDS epidemic because they linked the disease with homosexuality.[13]

This could explain why so few community-based programs for PLWAs are emanating from the African-American church. The earliest AIDS programs were conceived by coalitions of gay activists and by community leaders sympathetic to the suffering. Their responses forced, or perhaps shamed, churches into action.

RELIGION, POLITICS, RACE, AND SEXUAL ORIENTATION

Traditionally, the issue of homosexuality has not been discussed in the African-American community. This has not been an oversight. Rather, the African-American community has had more pressing concerns—racism chief among them. AIDS is just another burden.

"This is one more problem," said Alvin Poussaint, Harvard Medical School professor of clinical psychiatry, after a 1996 Harvard AIDS conference. "We've got crime, violence, teenage pregnancy, homelessness; now we've got AIDS."[14]

Just as feminists courted civil rights activists, gay-rights advocates have reached out to African-American leaders, drawing an analogy between gay and civil rights. Such efforts have met little success, but have won over some prominent civil rights leaders, including Reverend Jesse Jackson and Coretta Scott King, the widow of Martin Luther King Jr. Maverick preacher and political activist Al Sharpton has marched with ACT UP, a predominately gay AIDS group that employs civil disobedience to influence public policy. In an interview, Sharpton said he doesn't mind African-Americans and gays showing up on the same picket lines because he believes that AIDS should be combated universally.

"Some of the people in the AIDS movement did not know how to reach out and organize the black community," Sharpton noted. "Unlike the sixties and seventies, there has not been a coalition between some of the forces on the left and the black church. At one time the black leaders were the thermostat of public opinion. Now, we imitate others," he adds. "It is up to those who can put social policy on the agenda. I've not heard the cry we need to hear."[15]

Sharpton probably won't find many traditional African-American leaders willing to join him on the frontlines with ACT UP. Some mainline civil rights leaders are wary that gay issues could overshadow other concerns. Others believe sexual orientation and race are disparate issues. General Colin Powell, for example, is adamant that the armed forces should consider race and sexual orientation separately.

General Calvin Wallet, an African American who served in the Gulf War, went on record as saying, "I had no choice regarding my race when I was in my mother's womb. To compare my service in America's armed forces with the integration of avowed homosexuals is personally offensive to me."[16]

Many already view the African-American male as threatened or endangered. They point out that the white gay community has long been silent on the problems facing the African-American male and they will not allow gays to railroad their special interests without addressing the larger problems of the African-American community.

To enlist significant numbers of African-American churches in the battle against AIDS, The Balm in Gilead's Pernessa Seele walks a fine line between African-American and gay issues. To avoid controversy that might hinder the organization's effectiveness, for instance, The Balm in Gilead does not work with gay rights groups whose agenda is to push same-sex marriages on the church. The black AIDS community "must have the larger conversation and not go down this road where we get stuck on the homosexual theological issue," Seele insisted during an interview.

So volatile is the issue of homosexuality that the director of one African-American AIDS ministry in the nation's capital was allegedly told to never use the word "gay."

Given the gulf that exists between many African Americans and gays, it is easy to see why the white conservative establishment invited African-American ministers to join the religious right in opposing equal protection under the law for homosexuals. To put a wedge between the African-American and gay communities, the Traditional Values Coalition video, *Gay Rights, Special Rights,* contrasted a recent gay march on Washington with the historic 1963 March on Washington. In 1994, African-American ministers in Cincinnati, Ohio, embraced the video's conservative message and rallied the black community to help defeat a proposed gay rights ordinance. African-American leaders won over by these arguments fail to realize that conservatives use similar tactics to derail affirmative action.

Judicial decisions in cases dealing with gay rights issues have, upon occasion, blurred the line between church and state. In Richmond, Virginia, a federal court ruling upheld Virginia's anti-sodomy law in *Doe v. the City of Richmond.* The court cited passages from Leviticus as the rationale for its ruling. Several other states have borrowed biblical language to draft anti-sodomy laws. North Carolina, Virginia, Maryland, and Texas, for instance, base their anti-sodomy laws on the Book of Leviticus. Although the Constitution calls for strict separation of church and state, the boundary often gets obscured when it comes to laws governing homosexual lifestyles.

"AIDS' presumed African origin is also a barrier for some African Americans," said American Red Cross HIV/AIDS Coordinator Darlene Washington in a December 1995 *FDA Consumer* magazine article. "The disease was associated with Africa, and immediately, people said, 'I won't believe this. They are always blaming us for bad things. Why is Africa such a deep, dark place of teeming germs?'" (p. 4).[17]

While some African Americans resent reports that AIDS began in Africa and the designation of Haitian immigrants as a high-risk group, others suspect that the virus was engineered by whites to exterminate the African-American community. When the AIDs epidemic began sweeping minority communities in the 1980s, several conspiracy theories emerged. In 1990 the Southern Christian Leadership Conference surveyed 1,000 African-American churchgoers in five cities: Atlanta, Charlotte, Detroit, Kansas City, and Tuscaloosa. More than one-third thought AIDS was a form of racial genocide against African Americans, and another one-third believed the virus was produced in a germ warfare laboratory.[18]

Their suspicion is understandable considering the unethical treatment some African Americans suffered at the hands of medical researchers. In race memory, the AIDS virus and the Tuskegee Syphilis Study are forever linked. In the study, undertaken by the U.S. Public Health Department, nearly 400 African-American men who had syphilis were not truthfully diagnosed or administered penicillin when it was found to be the cure. The study was sanctioned by government physicians who relished the chance to chronicle the progression of the disease. The infamous study, which made virtual guinea pigs of its unknowing participants, persisted for more than forty years until a journalist exposed it in 1972. A 1974 lawsuit resulted in individual settlements of $37,500 each for the study's participants or their survivors.[19]

In May 1997, to heal racial scars, President Clinton offered an official apology for the study. At a White House ceremony, Herman Shaw, then ninety-five years old, accepted the president's apology for fellow study survivors. But, he stressed, "the wounds that were inflicted upon us cannot be undone."[20]

African-Americans' collective psyche still bears scars from the Tuskegee Study. Many African Americans are wary of legitimate medical research and government intervention that could result in advances in the treatment of diseases in blacks.

The Gospel Truth Is Still in the Closet

Although the African-American church has been a source of strength, hope, and enlightenment for the African-American community, it remains in the Dark Ages regarding AIDS and homosexuality. Because homosexuality is regarded by Western civilization as a taboo, most African-American churches have avoided discussing the issue or acknowledging the presence of gay members in its congregations. This stance marginalizes gay lifestyles and consigns homosexual AIDS victims to suffer alone. As a result, many homosexuals and lesbians die without the peace and compassion that should emanate from the church.

Former Howard University professor Ron Simmons suggests that gays have always been a part of the church community and have been involved in every aspect of church life, from playing the organ to teaching Sunday school. "As long as they did not openly display homosexual behavior," Simmons explained, "their presence was tolerated."[21]

Homosexuality is one of the African-American church's best kept secrets. Yet, the issue is right under its roof. In January 1996 in Delaware, there was a funeral for a gay member of the Ernest Davis Jr. Wilmington-Chester Mass Choir. In a 1996 interview, choir member Christopher Squires estimated that more than two dozen gospel musicians in the Wilmington, Delaware area died of AIDS from 1991 to 1994. Some choirs have lost so many members to the disease that they have been labeled "AIDS choirs."[22]

Gospel music is big business. An estimated forty million gospel records are sold each year. And a significant number of gays are involved in this segment of the music industry. The gospel music industry closely guards information about the sexual orientation of its artists. Some gay gospel performers even marry to conceal their lifestyles. And some choirs deny membership to openly gay artists. The African-American gospel music industry, which includes radio stations and television shows, takes great care to avoid the appearance of sanctioning or condoning homosexuality.

Thus, the spread of AIDS in gospel's underground homosexual subculture is widely rumored but seldom publicly acknowledged. This deadly silence stems from paranoia and theological disagreements about homosexuality in the African-American church.

In the African-American religious community, gay gospel artists get little respect or understanding—even as their recordings fly off store shelves. "Churches reverberate with their music, but condemn their lifestyles," said Reverend Yvette Flunder, pastor of City of Refuge United Church of Christ in San Francisco and former lead singer of the Walter Hawkins Love Center Choir. She noted with irony that African-American gospel artists appear at AIDS fund raisers in the white community, but rarely attend AIDS benefits in their own. In December 1996, however, Flunder, executive director of Ark of Refuge, a comprehensive AIDS ministry, broke the silence. She organized a major AIDS fundraiser in San Francisco that featured leading African-American gospel stars and acknowledged that AIDS was prevalent in the industry.

Because of the industry's silence on AIDS, Reverend Flunder thinks many musicians delay seeking treatment for fear of being discovered as HIV positive. She observed, "They go into seclusion just like sick animals to die. They are ashamed to go to places that can help."[23]

The mystery surrounding the death of Reverend James Cleveland epitomizes the shame. The gospel music legend and Los Angeles minister, who died in 1991, wrote more than 400 songs, recorded more than 100 albums, won sixteen gold records, and four Grammy awards. To keep up appearances, his death was officially attributed to heart disease, though it was rumored that AIDS was the actual cause.

His former foster son Christopher Harris allegedly contracted AIDS after years of sexual abuse by Cleveland. Harris sued Cleveland's estate. To keep the case out of the national media, Cleveland's family settled the case out of court for an undisclosed sum. Harris accuses the industry of denying both homosexuality and the AIDS issue. "They haven't dealt with the first part, so they are unable to deal with the second part."[24]

Meanwhile, AIDS is rampant in the African-American gospel community. Ministers preach funeral after funeral for artists who have succumbed to the disease. Too often, congregations and choirs bury the truth of homosexuality and AIDS along with its victims.

The African-American church has an obligation to help ease this pain because gay gospel artists are a vital part of the church's musical heritage. The church actually helped spawn the gospel music industry's early development by barring the genre from worship services. Of course, the church has since embraced gospel music. But it has yet to acknowledge the gay lifestyles that many gospel artists lead or the AIDS epidemic that threatens choirs, congregations, and the community.

The time has come for the African-American church to regard AIDS not as a sexual matter, but as a health crisis. This will not occur, though, until the African-American church's sexual theology comes into the modern age.

Chapter 4

Theology in the Time of AIDS

Black theology is the theology of a community whose daily energy must be focused on physical survival in a hostile environment.[1]

James Cone
A Black Theology of Liberation, 1990

Several events in this century have forced the Church to rethink its theology: Hiroshima, Auschwitz, and nuclear armament. These, however, are not the only modern crises that challenge theologians to find God in the midst of suffering. In 1987, Kevin Gordon presented a paper to the National Council of Churches, asking, "Is Theology Possible After AIDS?"[2] Indeed, the AIDS pandemic threatens to become the next Holocaust.

How do we do theology in the wake of AIDS? In an interview, Pernessa Seele insisted, "I don't think the church has to develop any kind of theology. The basis of the theology is the teaching of Jesus Christ. When we look at the ministry of Jesus, it's all there."[3]

In his book, *No Hiding Place,* Reverend Cecil Williams, pastor of San Francisco's Glide Memorial United Methodist Church, stated that the church should not debate theology when compassion is the prescription for pain.[4]

Others contend that the African-American church cannot address sexuality and AIDS until these issues have been explored in a theological context. In an interview, Reverend Carlton Veazey of the Religious Coalition for Reproductive Choice said, "For us to understand and dialogue on it [sexual orientation] will enable us to move on."[5]

Reverend Yvette Flunder, pastor of City of Refuge United Church of Christ in San Francisco and executive director of Ark of Refuge AIDS ministry, believes African Americans must overcome an oppressive theology in order to create community. "In this age of AIDS, the church ought to be more concerned . . . about the prima facie duty to do no harm. The church must remove the pejorative assumptions regarding [homosexuality] and provide equal access and equal opportunity for full participation."[6]

As a global crisis, AIDS compels the church to reexamine its theology and redefine our doctrines. In *The Black Experience in Religion*, C. Eric Lincoln noted, "For the first time the black church has the resources to engage in serious theological debate and to construct for itself a theology consistent with its needs" (p. 5).

At the millennium, the African-American church needs to address the AIDS epidemic. In the book, *Pastoral Theology: A Black Church Perspective*, James H. Harris observed that the African-American church "has historically balanced its Christ-centered worship and theology with a quest for social and political reform in the community" (p. 32).

Over the years, the African-American church has developed theologies to eradicate political and social oppression. The African-American church has always adapted to change at critical junctures in history. This is one of its strengths. The controversy surrounding the AIDS crisis, however, has immobilized some African-American church leaders who perceive conflict with church dogma.

A THEOLOGY FOR HEALING

Come to me all who are heavy laden and I will give you rest.

Matthew 11:28

If we do traditional theology, do we use an inductive model, moving from the human experience to make statements about

God, or a deductive model based on assumptions about God in relation to the human experience? The AIDS epidemic necessitates that we combine these models to help communities break the cycle of suffering and oppression.

In the African-American church, liberation theology addresses suffering and oppression by empowering people to challenge the status quo and realize their potential. Consequently, the African-American church has been the nation's conscience, midwifing the civil rights movement and working in the vineyard of justice and equality.

The church must reclaim the moral authority that made it a positive force in the midst of chaos. Liberation theology must continue to fight poverty, racism, and public policies that make minorities and the poor more likely to get HIV and more likely to die from AIDS. Further, liberation theology can help the African-American church overcome its own prejudices about those who are marginalized because of their lifestyles. Having felt the sting of racism, the African-American church must ensure that no group be made to suffer similar oppression.

The church must be a place where all people can come for healing. AIDS has caused brokenness, divisions, and despair. To alleviate the suffering, a theology for healing should facilitate reconciliation and affirm individual worth. Denial and rejection often occur within families living with AIDS. Some AIDS patients die alone because their family members abandon them. Fear of rejection also causes PLWAs to withdraw from the church and the community at a time when they most need comfort and compassion.

Reverend Alfonso Delany, pastor of Ebenezer United Methodist Church in Miami, witnessed this isolation in 1992 when he visited a Daytona hospital's AIDS ward. "There was a young man dying of AIDS who asked for us to call his mother. When she arrived, she turned her back on him and walked away. He was left to die alone with the knowledge that his mother rejected him," Delany recalled during an interview. "I knew then that we needed to start addressing the issue of AIDS from the pulpit."[7]

Jesus himself modeled a theology of healing by reaching out to the blind, lame, and sick—those who had been cast out. And people who were suffering sought out Jesus. Jesus used the Parable of the Prodigal Son to exemplify free will, love, and acceptance. Just as the Prodigal Son returned home, many PLWAs renew their ties to the church upon learning of their HIV status. Jesus allowed everyone to sit at the table. To facilitate healing of bodies, minds, and souls, the church must do the same. The church should accept PLWAs without preconditions.

In his 1992 memoir *No Hiding Place*, liberation theologist Cecil Williams wrote, "We need the church to respond with compassion—no other group can offer the Spirit, that's what the church has, and in Spirit and in truth the church can offer recovery and healing" (p. 216).

A THEOLOGY THAT RESPONDS TO SUFFERING

During my first year with the disease I nearly went crazy because I thought God was punishing me. I wondered why God would put a curse like AIDS on anyone. Later I realized that without God I wouldn't be able to make it.

Tanya, forty-four-year-old PLWA
Author interview, 1997

What does religion offer people when their backs are up against a wall? African Americans have had their backs against the wall of racism for more than 400 years. AIDS, however, has wrought a new kind of suffering.

Traditional interpretations of theology depict a God who is wrathful and vengeful toward sinners. For centuries, theologians have tried to justify why God allows suffering. In the early church, illness was viewed as a consequence of sin. Suffering was supposed to reconcile humankind with God. John Calvin taught that suffering came from the hand of God. Calvinists believed that everything that happened was providential, and that suffering challenged believers to respond positively to adversity.[8]

Those who suffer often blame themselves and their past actions for their ailments. To save others from similar suffering, some PLWAs speak about the risky behaviors that led to their infection.

During an interview, Steve, a homosexual who lives in an AIDS apartment complex, indicated that he identifies with Job. "I made the (lifestyle) choices and I have to live with the consequences. I had everything: a good job, lots of friends, a nice house. And then everything was taken away from me. My friends abandoned me. I lost my job and house and did not know what I was going to do. (But) I found strength in Christ," he attested. "This illness has brought me closer to God. I was brought up in the church and I got away from the teachings. If I can save someone's life by telling my story, then I have done something. No one deserves to have AIDS, no one."

In Romans 8:18, Paul put mortal suffering in spiritual perspective: "I consider that the sufferings of this present time are not worth comparing with the glory about to be revealed to us." Paul encourages the church at Rome to transcend earthly suffering and focus instead on the hope of eternal life.

As Jesus traveled to Jerusalem, a long-suffering woman made her way through the crowd. For years, she had had an issue of blood, a condition that Judaic law deemed unclean. Shunned by her community, she spent all her money on remedies, to no avail. On the crowded road to Jerusalem, her belief was confirmed that if she touched the hem of Jesus' garment, she would be healed. So strong was her faith that she drew His power into her, prompting Jesus to ask, "Who touched me?"

Enduring faith sometimes sustains PLWAs. Clarice, an ex-prostitute with a grown daughter, keeps the faith despite full-blown AIDS. "The doctors had given up on me," she remembers. "They told my sisters I was about to die. I did not claim AIDS as a part of my being. Yes, I have AIDS, but it does not have me. The power of God is what keeps me going and I am not afraid of death as a result. God knows where my heart is."

TOWARD A THEOLOGY OF SEXUALITY

There remains deeply entrenched in African-American churches a profoundly conservative theology of sexuality.

Michael Eric Dyson
Race Rules, 1996

Theologian James Cone contends that the African-American church has a rigid perspective on every issue except racism.

"One of the basic problems that has crippled the black church in the past," explained United Methodist minister Carlyle Fielding Stewart, "is the climate of repression which teaches people not to investigate, challenge, or critically appraise Scriptures or other religious tenets."[9]

For the most part, African Americans take the Bible at face value, particularly on sexual matters. As a result, African Americans—usually liberal on political issues—are decidedly conservative and judgmental when it comes to erotic desire and sexual identity.

This could be a legacy of slavery. The Protestant church taught enslaved Africans to cover their bodies in the daylight and hide behind closed doors in darkness. Thought beautiful in Africa, black bodies became objects of shame and guilt. In the hands of slave masters, the Bible was a tool to uphold white superiority. Blackness was connoted with sin and evil, and whiteness with goodness and virtue. Perverting religion, white slave masters discounted African-American minds and reviled African-American bodies. Systematically attacked for purposes of subjugation and control, African-American sexuality was not only deemed taboo, but bestial.

To refute these negative stereotypes, the African-American church's social, educational, and political missions aimed to uplift the community. African-American pastors preached the virtues of self-help and civic responsibility. Punctuated with gospel music, emotional sermons sometimes roused churchgoers to spiritual ecstasy, redefining worship as a whole-body experience. At the same time, Reconstruction-era African-American preachers demonized lust, adopting the Victorian values of the day. This rigid stance denied, repressed, and perverted healthy, African-American Christian sexuality.

Theologian Michael Eric Dyson believes an African-American theology of eroticism is needed to address the explosive sexuality fueling teen pregnancy, misogynistic rap lyrics, domestic abuse, male domination of church leadership, the spread of AIDS, and homophobia. For those of like minds, the AIDS epidemic presents an opportunity for the church to open dialogue on sexuality, from teen pregnancy to same-sex marriages.

Reverend Yvette Flunder, pastor of City of Refuge United Church of Christ in San Francisco argues that same-sex marriages would promote fidelity, reduce promiscuity, and stem the spread of AIDS. "(S)ame sex unions should not only be an acceptable practice in the Christian Church, but . . . are essential for the harmony of the church community where gay and lesbian parishioners are present,"[10] she asserted. Flunder charges that traditional church and denominational doctrines condemn gay lifestyles and thus marginalize gays and lesbians.

Bishop Carl Bean, pastor of Los Angeles' Unity Fellowship Church, also sanctions same-sex unions. A homosexual himself, he founded the congregation after being ostracized by the Baptist

Church. Multicultural in scope, Bean's brand of theology aims to liberate women, people of color, and homosexuals, encouraging parishioners to think and discern through human reason and experience. As a result, the church has attracted people—including transgender individuals—whom established churches have cast aside.

Mariah Britton, a youth minister at New York's Riverside Church, contends that new theologies are needed to address the sexuality of single individuals. "That old time religion is not going to be good enough for us," she said in a February 1998 interview. She believes scripture must be adapted to a contemporary cultural context, just as Paul's letters spoke directly to his times and audiences. "Paul was preaching out of the reality and urgency that he believed the Messiah was coming very soon," Britton explained. "Paul was a good Jew, and there were Deuteronomic and Levitical codes which predisposed him to women and marriage. Once you begin to interpret, you begin to break down those codes." For some believers, less than literal interpretations nullify the assurance of salvation, she observed.

Britton was one of several speakers at the National Black Religious Summit on Sexuality, held in June 1997 at Howard University School of Divinity. With the theme, "Breaking the Silence," the event, convened by Religious Coalition for Reproductive Choice, aimed to open dialogue on sexuality. The summit, however, was criticized for not including sexual orientation on its agenda. Even so, a groundbreaking position emerged from the event. The following consensus statement is intended to guide future work:

> Inasmuch as the Black church is the institutional pillar of the African-American community, historically providing moral support, spiritual renewal, and a venue for community-focused programs, we, the Black clergy, theologians, community, and youth leaders, realize our responsibility to address concerns about sexuality, including domestic vio-

lence, teen childbearing, and other matters of reproductive health, within the context of African-American communities of faith. With this in mind, we . . . the Clergy resolve to (1) support the development of a biblical and theological spirituality of sexuality; (2) continue to break the silence through an expanded agenda including all aspects of sexual orientation and expression inclusive of clergy sexual ethics; (3) continue to press and work for the training and education of church leadership and members on these issues, including getting our seminaries to produce leaders prepared to deal with these issues; and (4) to that end we will actively seek collaborative partnerships at local and national levels.

The Laity resolve to seek the Holy Spirit, to guide us in the dissemination of information in order to further educate and liberate the Black church community on a wide range of issues around sexuality. We further resolve to collaborate with pre-existing leadership and ministries in the church to develop and implement programs and activities to empower individuals to best live, that God is love and love is for everyone.

The Youth resolve to take the information we learned and give it back to the community through: self-defense classes, hot lines, advice columns, love clinics, rap sessions, counseling sessions, low-income nurseries, big brother/big sister relationships, and getting the church more involved in finding cures for sexually transmitted diseases. Further, we resolve to travel to other churches throughout the country to talk about what we learned at the Summit.[11]

Interestingly, the youth delegation was the only group to specifically target sexually transmitted diseases.

THE BIG TENT

For the African-American community, the church has had to be all things to all people. Each local congregation practices its own brand of theology that expresses indigenous experiences and desires. Research indicates that the more interaction people have with persons who are different from themselves, the more tolerant they become of diversity. When congregations shut out those who are different, they also close themselves off from God's creative power.

Liberation theology pitches a big tent, encompassing all who sojourn toward freedom, salvation, and wholeness. Having felt the sting of racism, the African-American church must ensure that no group be made to suffer similar oppression. As Jesus admonished in Matthew 25:40, "(J)ust as you did it to one of the least of these who are members of my family, you did it to me."

If African-American communities are to be freed from the scourge of AIDS, the church must answer God's call.

Chapter 5

What the Church Can Do

The African-American church has had to meet the issue head on, because AIDS has refused to go away. There have been just too many funerals for it to be ignored.[1]

Robert Fullilove, Associate Dean
Columbia University School of Health

Regardless of the size of its membership or budget, a church can impact at-risk populations and make a difference in the lives of people living with AIDS (PLWAs).

To determine needs and avoid duplication, churches interested in developing AIDS ministries should first identify and consult programs already in place in their communities. Representatives from AIDS agencies can be invited to the church to discuss their services. Churches can also invite PLWAs to tell their stories. As living witnesses, they can be valuable resources to churches in designing AIDS ministries.

One important consideration is the number of volunteers that a church can mobilize. The manpower requirements of a proposed ministry should not exceed the church's volunteer pool. Ministries must be staffed with enough volunteers to carry out long-term initiatives. Overworked volunteers are bound to burn out. When they do, ministries lose momentum and their clients suffer.

Father Russell Dillard pastors Washington's St. Augustine Catholic Church, which supports a regional feeding ministry.

Fifteen parishioners deliver meals to PLWAs. In a December 1997 interview, Dillard admitted, "People power is a problem. There are not a whole lot of people who want to get involved in an organized type ministry."

Reverend Seth Lartey, pastor of Goler Memorial A.M.E. Zion Church in Winston-Salem, North Carolina, added during a spring 1997 interview, "The majority of my church people are so busy just trying to maintain their middle-class lifestyles that they have no time or energy left to devote to causes that are not directly affecting them."

At San Francisco's Glide Memorial United Methodist Church, Reverend Cecil Williams calls parishioners to action with a theology that revisions the cross, one of Christianity's most sacred symbols. "The cross," he proclaimed, "will not save humanity—humanity will redeem the cross." For churches like Glide, AIDS ministries are a path to redemption.[2]

Regardless of whether churches develop AIDS ministries, their doors should be open to PLWAs. Congregations should greet PLWAs with open arms, offering solace and a sense of belonging. Through local media, church newsletters, and Sunday bulletins, churches can communicate their AIDS policies and send a message that they welcome PLWAs.

Even without direct participation by members, churches can provide meeting space—rooms underutilized during the week—for AIDS support groups. Support groups representing various congregations can meet at a centrally located church to share expenses. Some churches organize and facilitate support groups and grief counseling. Churches with a large facility and staff may even lend office space, equipment, and clerical assistance to local AIDS organizations.

Ministers have a responsibility to make their congregations aware of community needs. Through preaching and prayer, pastors create a climate of compassion and acceptance, and move parishioners to action.

"Jesus called the church into being to deal with those suffering," Reverend George McCray, pastor of Miami's Mount Tabor Missionary Baptist Church, stated in a February 1998 interview. "He touched those who had the greatest pain." The church should do no less.

As Wyatt Tee Walker, senior pastor of New York's Canaan Baptist Church of Christ, declared, "The African-American church must respond to the AIDS crisis if we claim Lordship in Christ."[3]

APPROACHES TO AIDS MINISTRY

PLWAs are a diverse group needing many services. Some churches run comprehensive AIDS ministries that address physical, emotional, spiritual, and financial needs. Others focus on one or more areas of need.

Delivery of services, however, can be a challenge. African Americans and other people of color have long been distrustful of public and private assistance efforts, especially when the programs are run by whites. Thus, African-American prevention and intervention programs may be able to reach some PLWAs that white-run efforts cannot. African-American churches, however, should be aware of common pitfalls: lack of funds, cultural insensitivity, community denial and distrust, and myths regarding AIDS transmission.

Regardless of their constituency, all church AIDS ministries are vital links in the care network. The following are some ways churches can get involved.

Spiritual Nurture

Of 300 studies on spirituality in scientific journals, the National Institute of Healthcare Research found that nearly three-fourths showed religion had a positive effect on health. Further, a

1988 study of 393 coronary patients at San Francisco General Hospital revealed that those who were prayed for had a lower incidence of congestive heart failure, pneumonia, and cardiac arrest and had less need for antibiotics than those who weren't.

Programs of spiritual nurture harness the power of prayer and show PLWAs that others empathize with them. All African-American churches can pray for PLWAs. That's the premise behind The Balm in Gilead's National Week of Prayer for the Healing of AIDS, an annual observance that involves more than 2,000 congregations nationwide. Denominational, ecumenical, and interfaith services periodically unite the community in prayer and healing. PLWAs, however, need prayer year round. Those at-risk, those infected and affected, and those who provide health care and social services to PLWAs need to be lifted up in prayers during worship services and prayer meetings. Bedside and hospital prayers are also needed. Churches can establish prayer groups and prayer chains and sponsor spiritual retreats for PLWAs and their families.

Support

Support ministries attend to physical and emotional needs, from nutrition and transportation to companionship. Large-scale feeding ministries, for example, use church kitchens to prepare meals and enlist volunteers to deliver the meals to PLWAs or to serve communal meals to PLWAs on site. Transportation networks help PLWAs run errands, visit doctors' offices, attend church, and take recreational outings.

Many PLWAs, particularly those who are homebound, long for community and for someone to listen and care. Buddy programs foster one-on-one relationships between church volunteers and PLWAs. Buddies phone and visit PLWAs on a regular basis. They may help PLWAs run errands, prepare meals, do housekeeping, and handle paperwork related to household expenses and medical insurance. Some PLWAs also need help with personal grooming. Others need advocates to negotiate financial and legal issues raised by the illness. These gestures mean a lot to PLWAs.

Church-run respite programs and adult day care centers also provide relief for caregivers. These initiatives enable caregivers to take much-needed breaks with the assurance that their loved ones are receiving quality care.

For the Children

To meet the needs of families, churches can open their day care, preschool, and recreational programs to children who are HIV positive. Strict adherence to safety procedures minimizes the infection risks to other children.

More children, however, have been orphaned by AIDS than infected with it. The CDC projects that as many as 125,000 children could be orphaned by the year 2000. Some churches work with foster care and adoption agencies to find prospective placements for HIV-positive children and children orphaned by AIDS. In many cases involving African-American children, grandparents and aunts assume care. Custodial grandparents, some of whom have serious medical problems of their own, need additional support. Congregations can offer financial aid to grandparents faced with caring for AIDS orphans, provide transportation for medical visits, counseling, and support groups. Some churches also provide volunteers and funding for orphanages and children's homes that serve children living with AIDS.

Housing

Housing programs are designed to meet the needs of AIDS patients who become homeless or too sick to continue living independently. The living situations that housing programs offer range from hospices and long-term care facilities to community-based apartment buildings and group homes. Like any real estate venture, AIDS housing programs are expensive to develop and manage. Consequently, few churches operate such programs.

Financial Aid

As their health declines, many PLWAs become unable to work. Faced with lost income and mounting medical bills, some PLWAs lack money for rent or mortgage, food, transportation, and other expenses. Church benevolence and voucher programs can help with financial emergencies.

Fund-Raising

Churches that have no direct involvement with PLWAs can help fund nonprofit groups and church ministries that target PLWAs and high-risk groups. Churches can earmark special offerings and hold fund-raisers to benefit AIDS ministries, agencies and organizations.

Street Outreach

Through Street Outreach, church volunteers target high-risk groups in the community. Street Outreach may promote AIDS awareness, HIV testing, condom use, or needle exchange. Some churches distribute AIDS literature. Some administer HIV testing, while others refer individuals to health agencies. Through condom distribution programs, Street Outreach volunteers encourage members of high-risk groups to practice safe sex.

Some church volunteers exchange drug users' dirty syringes for needles that have been sterilized with bleach. Opposed by the federal government, needle exchange programs are, nevertheless, advocated by the National Medical Association, the National Black Caucus of State Legislators, and the National Black Nurses Association. Six independent studies show that needle exchange programs stop AIDS transmission without increasing drug use. One-third of pediatric AIDS cases and the majority of HIV infections in African-American females are injection related. Though controversial, these programs are much needed.

Advocacy

The voices of African Americans need to be heard in local, state, and national discussions on HIV/AIDS. The African-American church can use its influence to shape AIDS public policy and funding decisions. Government and foundation support for AIDS programs targeting African Americans is much less than it should be given the disproportionately high rate of AIDS infection among African Americans. Similarly, women, children, minorities, and the poor often lack adequate access to treatment. Concerned churches can lobby for more services for underserved PLWAs and high-risk populations. Advocacy efforts include contacting elected officials, public health agencies, nonprofit organizations, civil rights groups, and schools to increase awareness of the epidemic and the needs of PLWAs.

Other Initiatives

Many church-based AIDS ministries also focus on prevention education and pastoral care. These initiatives will be discussed in detail in subsequent chapters.

Chapter 6

Teaching What We Preach: AIDS Prevention Education

Sex education is all about values. What better place to teach values than the church?[1]

Henry Foster, MD
Senior Advisor to the President
on Teen Pregnancy Reduction
and Youth Issues

TO TEACH OR NOT TO TEACH?

A 1996 Gallup Poll revealed that teenagers were less afraid of getting AIDS in 1995 than in 1991. This despite CDC reports that AIDS is the leading cause of death among African Americans aged fifteen to twenty-four. Though today's teens have less fear of infection, they continue to believe that sex education is the best way to stop the spread of AIDS.

Toward that end, many public schools offer AIDS education and sex education curricula. Some churches adamantly oppose sex education and condom distribution. But most African-American churches have been absent from the pedagogy and the debate, at a time when more and more schools are not only teaching sex education but integrating character education into their courses of study. Uniquely qualified to put sexuality in a religious context, the African-American church must lend its voice to the discourse.

From the founding of colleges to mid-week bible study, teaching has always been a function of the African-American church. AIDS-prevention education, however, is unfamiliar territory for most churches.

Beyond advocating marital fidelity, most churches would rather not broach the private and complex subject of sex. In fact, many African-American churches all but deny that sex is central to our makeup as human beings. Not surprising, many churches are reluctant to discuss the issues related to AIDS-prevention education.

"Not all churches want to deal in detailed prevention education," said theologian Wardell Payne in a January 1998 interview. "They have a problem with explicit discussions . . ." he explained, "(and) the perception that you're sanctioning behavior which should be banned according to the teaching of the church."[2]

This poses a moral and spiritual dilemma for many African-American churches. But AIDS-prevention education also presents an opportunity for churches to impart religious values that will ultimately save lives.

WHO NEEDS TO KNOW?

Before administering a church-wide education program, church leaders must first be trained. This includes the pastor, staff, Sunday school teachers, and others involved in the church's educational ministries. Experienced HIV/AIDS educators suggest that five to six sessions be allotted for in-depth training. If one day-long session is held, follow-up will be needed.

Among the topics that should be covered are: AIDS statistics in the African-American community, sexual intimacy, abstinence, monogamy, intravenous drug use and needle sharing, care for PLWAs, community resources, condom use, and public policy. The training should not only inform but confront participants' attitudes about the disease. This will help prospective facilitators shake the prejudices that may turn off those they hope to reach.

People of all ages and genders can benefit from prevention education. The rise in AIDS rates among older adults, for example, suggests that this group lacks knowledge of risk factors and transmission modes. While some churches offer AIDS-prevention education to their congregations, others target at-risk groups in their communities: intravenous drug users, homosexuals, women, adolescents, or prison inmates.

Prevention-education efforts targeting African-American women are sorely needed. Not only are women themselves vulnerable to infection through intravenous drug use and heterosexual contact, but they also risk passing the virus to their unborn child(ren).

Older adults also need prevention education. AIDS is on the rise among seniors, many of whom are unaware that they are at risk.

Prevention specialists caution that programs that work for one population may not be effective for other populations. There is no one-size-fits-all curriculum.

WHAT SHOULD THE CHURCH TEACH?

Prevention education is most effective when it is explicit, interactive, and age appropriate. Education efforts targeting African Americans should also be culturally sensitive: acknowledging the psychology of sexual racism, promoting positive global images of African Americans, and integrating positive views of sexuality within the framework of the culture. Howard Stevenson, a professor at the University of Pennsylvania, stressed that empowerment should be a key focus of prevention-education programs targeting African Americans.[3] In addition, African themes and values can help promote healthy lifestyles.

Before launching prevention-education efforts, churches should contact schools, health agencies, and community organizations to determine what existing prevention programs cover. AIDS education programs should highlight statistics, dispel myths, alleviate fears, and, most important, explain prevention methods. To give a face to the disease, invite PLWAs to share firsthand experiences during the training. Personal narratives convey the magnitude of the disease and provoke discussion. Storytelling, an African-American oral tradition, helps participants feel at home and makes them more receptive to the training's lifesaving message.

The African-American church is not of one mind on AIDS prevention education. The sheer number of denominations and doctrines reduces the likelihood that any single prevention-education model will suit the needs of every local church. That doesn't stop some folks from trying, though. With funding from the Kaiser Family Foundation, The Balm in Gilead, which mobilizes and trains churches to combat AIDS, is designing the first Sunday school curriculum on the disease.

Abstinence from premarital and extramarital sex and from drug use should form the core of what churches teach. Beyond these basics, churches must develop curricula compatible with their theology. The Bible does not directly address sexually transmitted diseases (STDs) such as AIDS. The church need not ignore current realities: premarital sex, teenage pregnancy, sexual promiscuity, homosexuality, rising heroin use, the increase in heterosexual AIDS transmission, and the spread of AIDS among prison populations. The church should provide comprehensive information so those who do not abstain know other effective prevention methods.

Reverend Mariah Britton, associate minister of youth at New York's Riverside Church, noted that people make sexual choices with or without the blessing of the church or the state. Britton, who contended that premarital chastity denies natural urges, believes churches need a new ethic to address the sexual issues facing singles. "In this climate where your selection of mate could be your death sentence," she said, "it is critical that the church speak with knowledge and compassion about condoms, contraceptives, and STDs."[4]

The AIDS epidemic signals a state of emergency and calls for crisis intervention. This compels the church to adopt radical approaches that may initially appear to run counter to its theology. In the book *Race Rules*, Michael Eric Dyson wrote, "The black church should lay off the hard line approach on teenage sexual activity. Sure, it must preach abstinence first. It should also preach and teach safe sex, combining condoms and common sense" (p. 94).[5]

More effective than preaching at teenagers about abstinence are forums that enable them to ask, and get answers to, their questions about human sexuality, relationships, drugs, and AIDS. Though parents and pastors espouse abstinence, the media projects contradictory images and messages. And some teens use intimacy to alleviate feelings of alienation and low self-esteem.

AIDS prevention education should affirm individual worth and help youth make wise choices. Teens should learn Biblical and theological foundations, the virtues of abstinence, and prevention methods. To reach youth, adult educators must be committed to growth and understanding. They must establish trust and keep confidences, but not dangerous or illegal secrets. Children will undoubtedly ignore some of the lessons they learn. But Proverbs 22:6 assures, "Train children in the right way, and when they are old they will not stray."

In 1996, Second Baptist Church in Perth Amboy, New Jersey, convened a seminar for teenage girls called "My Body, God's Temple." Facilitators found that sex was not foremost on the teens' minds. They were more interested in talking about relationships and self-respect. One participant said the program showed her that the women in the church cared. This message alone could promote healthy attitudes among adolescent girls.

While youth need prevention education, parents also need guidance in exploring human sexuality and talking about AIDS with their children. Data indicate that peers and the media are the primary source of information on STDs for 89 percent of U.S. teens. The other eleven percent get most of their STD information from their parents. The church doesn't even figure in the equation.

Training sessions are not the only way to disseminate AIDS prevention information. Religious, recreational, and cultural events such as revivals, health fairs, African-inspired rites-of-passage programs, and AIDS quilt displays have been utilized to raise consciousness and promote testing and prevention. Churches can also enlist the nation's 150 gospel radio stations, which reportedly reach 90 percent of African-American households, to spread the word about prevention. Such outreach efforts are crucial, since the church enjoys only marginal attendance among some at-risk groups.

A Nigerian proverb states, "It takes a whole village to educate a child." When it comes to AIDS-prevention education, the church's teachings are essential.

Chapter 7

Pastoral Care
for People Living with AIDS

The resident psychologists are the pastors and the mothers and fathers of the church. Every person brings their own couch and if they listen, the answers are given without having to pay $150 an hour.[1]

Frank Reid, Pastor
Bethel A.M.E. Church
Baltimore, Maryland

BETWEEN THE LINES OF SERMONS

In the African-American church, much pastoral counseling takes place between the lines of Sunday sermons. Steeped in the oral tradition, African-American sermons encourage parishioners to keep the faith despite hardship, heartache, and injustice. From the pulpit, healing words, punctuated with poignant stories and sage advice, help churchgoers bear up under oppression and beat back depression.

In African tribal culture, the priest and healer were one, overseeing ritual and medicine. Today, the African-American pastor is still called to offer spiritual healing. In his book *No Hiding Place*, Reverend Cecil Williams, minister of liberation at San Francisco's Glide Memorial United Methodist Church, observed, "Coming to church for help is acceptable behavior for black people" (p. 204).

There is no other institution or organization better equipped to provide spiritual care. Ideally, pastoral care is perpetual, beginning before birth and extending beyond death. As the saying goes, "From the moment we are born, we begin to die." Diseases such as HIV/AIDS, with accompanying physical, emotional, and spiritual pain, are part of that continuum.

Pastors are not only expected to counsel parishioners on how to live but how to die as well. PLWAs need pastoral care that liberates them from the fear of death, frees them to live, and strengthens them to face uncertainty. That's a tall order in a society that often shuns issues of death and dying. To make matters worse, many pastors are ill-prepared or too puritanical to deal with the complexities of HIV/AIDS. A study by C. Eric Lincoln and Lawrence Mamiya found that less than two-thirds of African-American clergy hold bachelor's degrees and less than 80 percent have had any seminary training.[2] Most seminaries require only one course in pastoral counseling. This infers that a significant number of pastors are insufficiently trained to counsel PLWAs.

Lack of educational credentials, however, should not be an obstacle to compassionate pastoral care. HIV/AIDS education offered through public health agencies and nonprofit organizations can help pastors gain knowledge and develop sensitivity regarding the complex issues facing PLWAs, their families, and caretakers.

The preacher's attitude helps shape the congregation's outlook on such social and health issues as HIV/AIDS. Consequently, trained pastors increase their congregations' HIV/AIDS awareness and dispel misconceptions that breed fear, denial, and condemnation.

From the pulpit, the pastor also models compassion. If a pastor depicts AIDS as punishment for sin and PLWAs as unclean, parishioners will be less likely to reach out to them. Further, PLWAs will be reluctant to confide in the pastor and may stay away from the church at a time when they need spiritual support more than ever.

In focus groups PLWAs discussed their relationships with God and the church. David (not his real name), a thirty-two-year-old married man living with AIDS, attested, "I am dealing with a crisis now, and I don't want to leave here without making peace with God."

Kathy, a forty-one-year-old single woman living with AIDS, hesitates to reveal her health status to the church. "The church's attitude," she said, "makes me not be open. Church is like family. I sometimes feel like I should open up to them, but other times I want to withdraw because I don't want them to know. I was brought up in the church. I sing in the choir. I love my church a lot. But I can't be open. I feel like the church would condemn me."

Pastoral counseling should work to alleviate this isolation, convey love and acceptance, and reconcile PLWAs to their spiritual roots. In so doing, it can restore wholeness and emotional balance.

COMMON SENSE AND UNCOMMON LOVE

PLWAs need to hear of God's grace, love, and forgiveness, so they can find peace with God.

Reverend Don Nations, an HIV/AIDS instructor and pastor of Lemonia Village United Methodist Church in Brandon, Florida, believes pastoral care can offer assurance to PLWAs by conveying ten core beliefs:

> God loves all of us.
> God will draw near to us.
> God offers forgiveness.
> God is with us.
> God brings good into our life.
> God gives us purpose.
> God gives us strength.
> God's gifts are peace, hope, and joy.
> God takes the side of the poor, the sick, and the oppressed.
> God never gives up on us.[3]

There is only one way to minister to any person—with love and compassion. Pastors should offer counsel, comfort, and hope.

Carolyn McCrary, an assistant professor at the Interdenominational Theological Seminary, said the pastoral counselor's role is
"to stand at the foot of the cross patiently waiting and working
with persons as they externalize, express, expel, and re-internalize
or gather together dimensions of themselves that heal toward
wholeness."[4]

Counseling itself should also be culturally specific. According to
Edward Wimberly, also a professor at the Interdenominational
Theological Seminary, pastors can assist African Americans by
exploring prehistoric African archetypes that instill pride, affirm
identity, and validate self-worth; using storytelling to build intimacy
and trust; examining stories and myths—Biblical and otherwise—
that clients identify with; modeling emotional responses through
self-disclosure; and stressing the importance of support systems.[5]

The following guidelines for pastoral care to PLWAs incorpo-
rate common sense and uncommon love.

Do Not Ask PLWAs How They Got Infected

When people have common illnesses such as cancer or heart
disease, we don't inquire how they got sick. Thus, why should we
feel that an AIDS diagnosis entitles us to pry into a person's past?
PLWAs are usually more concerned with the present and future
than with the past. PLWAs can not change their past, but they can
find serenity in learning to accept it. Lifestyle issues surrounding
modes of AIDS transmission may need to be discussed at some
point in counseling, but not at the outset. The first meeting, when
the pastor learns the person's HIV status, sets the tone for all future
visits or interactions. The pastor's initial reaction will in large part
determine the quality of care he or she will be able to provide. The
first meeting is a time for compassion not interrogation.

Avoid Blaming the Victim

When Jesus was expected to render a death sentence to the
adulterous woman (John 8:11), he stunned the crowd by offering

forgiveness instead. All human beings have taken risks and been spared the consequences. It is hypocritical to blame those who suffer the consequences of their acts. Plus, guilt slows healing. The self-righteous and judgmental render themselves ineffective.

Be Compassionate

Jesus always showed compassion, even when He commanded individuals to change their ways. Compassion involves withholding judgment and focusing instead on needs. It is conveyed through gentleness, kindness, acceptance, and love. It means being a channel of God's grace and aiding those who are hurting.

Face Fears About HIV/AIDS

Some pastors still believe the myths about AIDS transmission. To make matters worse, they perpetuate these misconceptions from the pulpit, causing the church to reject and neglect PLWAs. Ignorance and prejudice prevent pastors and congregations from reaching out to those in need of help. It is crucial that ministers get the facts about AIDS to dispel fears and remove barriers to interaction and involvement.

Emphasize Life and Offer Hope

Death is a fact of life for PLWAs and for everyone else as well. A counseling session with a PLWA is not the place to dwell on death. Rather, the focus should be on living abundantly and restoring hope. Jesus offers hope that God gives life meaning and promises eternity. Regardless of their prognosis, PLWAs have much living left to do. HIV/AIDS is not an immediate death sentence. Some PLWAs have survived for more than a decade. New medications, such as protease inhibitors, have prolonged the life expectancy of PLWAs. New treatments are being discovered, and a cure may eventually be found. Further, studies show that prayer itself is a powerful medicine.

Let the Individual Set the Agenda for Discussion

Efforts to control or direct the conversation can undermine the counseling session and sabotage even the best intentions. People tend to withdraw from those who seek to control them. Particularly during the early stages of the relationship, the PLWA needs to dictate the topics of discussion. Refrain from demanding that the PLWA repent, notify partners or family members, and accept death. Such demands will ultimately prove counterproductive.

Maintain Confidentiality

Like doctor/patient and lawyer/client relationships, the relationship between pastor and parishioner requires confidentiality. Do not betray a person's trust by discussing their case with anyone, including spouses, family members, friends, and other church leaders. It's not easy for someone to reveal his or her HIV status, particularly to authority figures such as pastors. Revealing one's secret involves baring one's soul. Thus, disclosure increases vulnerability and takes incredible courage. Breaking confidentiality can result in irreparable damage to the relationship between pastor and parishioner.

Affirm Individual Worth

God extends His grace to all people, regardless of physical infirmity. One of the most cherished Christian beliefs is that we are all made in the image of God. In His eyes, all human beings are equals, possessing great dignity and eternal worth. He calls all people to a life filled with power, love, joy, and service to others. That message of love is inherent in the Gospel.

Express Emotions Freely

HIV/AIDS provokes concerns about life-and-death issues. By confronting these issues, pastoral care brings strong emotions to the surface. Pastors need to be in touch with their own feelings about these issues. But they must not let their own feelings of fear, anxiety, and pity temper their responses to PLWAs. Nor should they suppress their emotions. Pastors should feel free to be themselves—to cry, laugh, and express other emotions—when visiting PLWAs.

Recognize the Importance of Physical Touch

Many people still fear physical contact with PLWAs. This fear usually results from misconceptions regarding transmission modes and from stigmas associated with homosexuals and heroin users, high-risk groups for contracting the disease. Failure to touch, however, implies the withholding of emotions and acceptance. Pastors must overcome prejudice and fear to administer touch and connect with PLWAs. For many parishioners, the laying on of hands is the key to spiritual healing.

Recognize the Stages of Grief

PLWAs go through several stages of grief: shock, denial, anger, bargaining, depression, and acceptance. There is no set schedule for any stage, and people often bounce back and forth between stages. The pastor's job is not to make grief go away or to hasten the progression from one stage of grief to another. Rather, pastors should help PLWAs wrestle with their present stage and lend support during difficult times.

Know the Psychosocial Issues Surrounding AIDS

PLWAs face complex issues, including social isolation, rejection by friends and family, prolonged illness, uncertainty about the future, prejudice, reproductive decisions, guilt, and grieving. Pastors must recognize these issues before they can help PLWAs work through them. Further, pastors need to educate and mobilize their congregations and communities to respond supportively.

Honor Others' Spiritual Expressions, Beliefs, and Experiences

Recognize that religion and spirituality vary from person to person and that people experience and respond to God in different ways. God uses a different voice to speak to each person and touches each person in a unique way. The structure of organized religion is no substitute for true compassion. Pastors should not assume that they have insight into peoples' spirituality or that PLWAs are not spiritual. Nor should pastors presume to have insight into peoples' spirituality. The pastor is merely a guide to help parishioners find their own path on their faith journey.

Resist the Inclination to Say, "I know how you feel"

No matter how much one may empathize with another, no one can fully understand how another person feels. People respond to the same situations and experiences in different ways. Painful testimonies sometimes leave pastors at a loss for words. The comment, "I know how you feel," sounds hollow and false. More appropriate responses include, "I'm sorry"; "I hear what you're saying"; "How can I help?"; "Tell me how that makes you feel"; or "I'm here to listen." Sometimes a nonverbal response works best; when words do not suffice, a gentle touch or sincere embrace shows caring.

Understand That Pastoral Care to PLWAs Can Be a "Long Haul"

People who are HIV positive can take years to develop the symptoms of AIDS, and the life expectancy of PLWAs is increasing each year. For PLWAs, the disease poses ongoing challenges. Each family member will have different needs. HIV/AIDS is not a problem that can be resolved in a one-hour counseling session.

Pastoral care for PLWAs takes time, patience, and rapport. The pastor's role is not to have all the answers but to be present and lend support through suffering and grief. In so doing, pastors meet God in others. Through pastoral care, pastors confront their own emotions, prejudice, and spirituality. This opens them up to experiencing the conversion that results from personal growth.

Admit When Issues Are Beyond Your Expertise and Make Appropriate Referrals

Pastors are not health care professionals, social workers, or lawyers. We cannot address all of the issues surrounding AIDS. Don't hesitate to say, "I don't know," and to refer parishioners to experts and to resource agencies within the community.

WHO NEEDS PASTORAL CARE?

Pastoral care not only benefits people infected with AIDS but also those whose lives are affected by the disease—family members, partners, and caregivers. It hurts to witness a loved one's physical decline and to know that death is imminent. Emotionally, physically, and spiritually taxing, caretaking inevitably becomes a burden. Not surprisingly, this stress sometimes leads to burnout.

Yet, the needs of caregivers are often dwarfed by the needs of those they care for. But caregivers' and families' needs are just as urgent. In fact, these individuals' feelings and actions color how the infected persons feel about themselves and their futures. That's why it's important for pastoral care to embrace families and caregivers.

How can a pastor minister to the diverse needs of so many people? In addition to one-on-one counseling, pastors may also need to consider organizing and leading HIV/AIDS support groups for persons infected and affected by the disease. By bringing together people who face similar challenges, support groups help reduce the isolation often associated with HIV/AIDS. Support groups can also help facilitate the healing of broken relationships. Consequently, support groups can restore a sense of community.

In an interview, Robert (not his real name) discussed his participation in a support group. He had been married for several years when the health department alerted him that he may have been exposed to HIV during a premarital relationship. The news that he tested HIV positive was a blow to Robert and his family. Fortunately, a sympathetic pastor helped Robert and his wife deal with the emotional issues brought about by the discovery. Their minister also referred them to a support group. Robert said he and his wife drew strength from this setting. Involvement with other PLWAs, he said, prepared them for the changes ahead.

THE DANGERS OF DENIAL

Denial is a stage of grief, a natural defense against pain and suffering. Pastors and caregivers must allow for this reaction. Denial manifests itself in several ways. Some PLWAs stop taking their medicines because they don't believe they need it. Others may continue behaviors that put others at risk, such as unsafe sex or needle-sharing. Pastors should extend spiritual comfort, so PLWAs will confront their fears and get beyond the denial that may endanger others.

Jesus assured his followers that He would be with them until the end. He reached out to the hurting, never ceasing to participate in their suffering with his physical presence. The secular world is unpredictable and often cruel. Pastoral care reminds PLWAs that the community of faith embodies God's love, a constant source of peace and hope.

Chapter 8

In the Trenches:
African-American AIDS Ministries

. . . the best-connected network I know is the church. It's not good enough to be a haven for the saved; I'm going to ask them to be a hospital for the sick and the sinners.[1]

Former U.S. Surgeon General Joycelyn Elders
Butler University, Indianapolis, Indiana, 1994

In the 1980s, the Centers for Disease Control (CDC) instituted a Faith Initiative. This initiative recognizes churches' vast constituency, political influence, stability, volunteer orientation, charity, and potential as change agents. The Initiative's stated mission is: "To support and foster HIV prevention activities and partnerships involving faith communities to promote an integrated and comprehensive response to the HIV/AIDS epidemic . . . "[2]

The CDC carries out its mission through education, information, marketing and material development, technical assistance, network and partnership development, and research and evaluation. The CDC also seeks common ground between faith communities and public health agencies. Prior to 1995, none of the Faith Initiative's national partners had an African-American focus. In response to disproportionately high infection rates in the African-American community, the initiative has since forged relationships with The Balm in Gilead and the Congress of National Black Churches. The CDC urges denominations and congregations to determine their own best responses to HIV/AIDS, based on their theological beliefs and principles.

That's just what some African-American churches and religious are doing. The leadership and ministries highlighted in this chapter represent the diverse efforts being mounted in communities across the country. Unless otherwise cited, this information was gleaned from surveys, interviews, and organizational publications.

ECUMENICALS TAKE THE LEAD

Southern Christian Leadership Conference

Co-founded by Martin Luther King Jr., the Southern Christian Leadership Conference (SCLC) was the first mainline civil rights group to address the AIDS issue. SCLC/Women, an adjunct of the Atlanta-based SCLC, developed the National AIDS Awareness Program. Under the leadership of Evelyn Lowery, SCLC/Women trained ministers and parishioners to administer educational and prevention workshops in local churches. The initiative also helped participating churches get to the root of homophobia and become more tolerant of gay men and lesbians. In 1991, the organization held a convention on HIV/AIDS and the church—the same weekend that basketball star Earvin "Magic" Johnson disclosed his HIV-positive status. The program is now defunct.[3]

Congress of National Black Churches

In 1992 the Washington-based Congress of National Black Churches (CNBC) held a groundbreaking meeting on "Theological Perspectives on Sexuality in the African-American Community." The meeting, which CNBC dubs its annual consultation, tackled sensitive topics—among them AIDS, homosexuality, sexually transmitted diseases, birth control, and male-female relationships. The previous year, CNBC cosponsored a conference on substance abuse which led to its National Anti-Drug

Campaign funded by the U.S. Department of Justice. The campaign eventually expanded its scope to include AIDS.[4]

By 1997, CNBC saw the need for a more focused AIDS effort. The National African-American Religious Summit on HIV/AIDS was held in conjunction with the organization's consultation on "Healing Streams." With funding from the Centers for Disease Control and Prevention, the summit provided a forum to discuss AIDS ministries and to determine how the church should respond.

The Balm in Gilead

In 1989 Pernessa Seele, then a newcomer to New York, went door to door enlisting African-American churches to join in the Harlem Week of Prayer for the Healing of AIDS. She conceived the event after losing her church choir director to AIDS and witnessing the deaths of AIDS patients at Harlem Hospital where she worked. The African-American church, she said, was noticeably absent from those sickrooms. The week of prayer gave birth to The Balm in Gilead, a New York-based nonprofit organization, which remains in the forefront on the AIDS issue in the black community.

In 1992 the prayer event evolved into the Black Church National Day of Prayer for the Healing of AIDS. Now known as the Black Church Week of Prayer for the Healing of AIDS, the program focuses aims to soften worshipers' attitudes and hearts regarding HIV/AIDS. The nationwide event calls African-American clergy and laypersons to action by providing prevention education and encouraging compassion for people living with AIDS. Observed by more than 2,000 African-American churches, the program aims to spark mobilization, AIDS prevention education, and pastoral care efforts.

Participating churches, called Certified Network Partners, receive worship resources, educational materials, ongoing technical assistance, support services, and evaluation. The Balm in Gilead holds a semiannual national training and technical assistance conference. Required training for Partners covers African-American theology and HIV/AIDS, mobilization strategies, program planning and implementation, public relations, financial management and fund raising, and coalition building. Partners must also assemble a planning team including representatives from the church, media, business, community agencies, AIDS advocacy groups, public health departments, schools, colleges and seminaries, persons living with AIDS, and the black gay and lesbian community.[5]

In February 1994, the organization convened the First African-American Religious Leaders Summit on HIV/AIDS at the White House. During the summit, forty prominent Black ministers signed a "Declaration of War on HIV/AIDS," vowing to battle AIDS through prevention education, counseling, advocacy, sermons and prayers.[6]

Ten major African-American church denominations and caucuses have endorsed The Balm in Gilead's mission to educate and mobilize African-American church communities to develop AIDS ministries. The organization has received a research grant from the CDC and funding from the Kaiser Family Foundation to design the first Sunday school curriculum on AIDS. The organization receives support from the Ford Foundation, Public Welfare Foundation, New York Community Trust, United Methodists Church Division of Women, and Black Presbyterians. Small contributions also come from individual churches.

AIDS Advocacy in African-American Churches Project

The AIDS Advocacy in African-American Churches Project (AAAACP) is a national constituency group of African-American clergy and other laypeople who provide care and compassion to PLWAs. The organization promotes physical and spiritual health and wholeness in the midst of suffering, guilt, and shame felt by PLWAs. AAAACP aims to increase the number of local, regional, and national church-based AIDS ministries and to combat the stigma of AIDS through culturally specific education and training. The organization also publicizes the efforts of African-American religious leaders in the fight against AIDS.

National African-American Church AIDS Council

In 1989 several African-American churches formed the National Black Church AIDS Council. The Council sought ways to disseminate AIDS information without compromising religious teachings and values. Reverend Joseph Davis, a United Methodist minister in Eutaw, Alabama, was the Council's first chair. From 1989 to 1990, the organization sponsored five regional conferences that aimed to establish a national training model and build alliances among pastors and health care workers. The council also planned to teach pastoral counseling to help ministers assist PLWAs. The Council, which eventually shifted its focus, is now known as the National Black Church Family Council.

MODEL AIDS MINISTRIES

Nation of Islam Ministry of Health and Human Services

The Nation of Islam (NOI) has taken a more aggressive and comprehensive approach to AIDS than other African-American denominations. During a July 1997 health forum sponsored by Congressman Louis Stokes (D-OH), Abdul Alim Muhammad, MD, NOI minister of health and human services, detailed a nine-point program.[7] He contends that:

1. African Americans must acknowledge the toll AIDS has taken in their community and its potential as a species-threatening epidemic.
2. HIV education in the African-American community should highlight AIDS mortality statistics among people of color in

the United States and worldwide, the transmission of AIDS by formerly incarcerated males to African-American women, and the spread of AIDS among young adults.

3. Widespread HIV testing and on-the-spot diagnosis is necessary to identify infected individuals and make them aware of their responsibility to prevent the spread of AIDS.

4. The African-American community needs to develop a comprehensive network of compassionate caring to reduce the suffering, pessimism, and hopelessness that attend an HIV-positive diagnosis. Pre- and posttesting counseling for HIV-positive individuals should involve health and social service professionals, clergy, community activists, and laypersons.

5. PLWAs in the African-American community and in developing countries lack the financial resources to obtain expensive treatments such as protease inhibitors. These communities need to be given access to lower-cost alternative therapies.

6. The government should increase funding for HIV research involving African-American researchers, institutions, and patients.

7. Infrastructure development is urgently needed. The nation's 22,000 African-American doctors can only offer a doctor-to-patient ratio of one physician to every 1,500 African-American patients—far too low to ensure proper health maintenance. More health facilities are also needed in the African-American community. And small community-based AIDS organizations need technical assistance and capacity-building resources.

8 and 9. AIDS must be regarded as a global, species-threatening pandemic requiring the human race to rise above ethnic, cultural, economic, political, and geographic barriers to form against a common foe.

The centerpiece of NOI's AIDS ministry is the Abundant Life Clinic, an urban health care facility located in a low-income housing development in northeast Washington, DC. Since 1991, the clinic has specialized in the treatment of HIV/AIDS. The clinic focuses on natural alternative treatments, especially a low-dose, oral alpha interferon therapy developed in Kenya. Alpha interferon is a natural substance produced by the human immune system to combat infection. Commonly known as "kemron" or "Immunex," the treatment reportedly resolved the symptoms of AIDS in some patients. Further, treatment costs average $800 a year, compared to $10,000 a year for AZT, a widely used synthetic drug. Clinical trials sponsored by the National Institutes of Health began in 1996 at sixteen participating sites, including three historically black medical institutions—Howard University Medical Center, Meharry Medical College, and King/Drew Medical Center. After about one year, the trials ended inconclusively. The Abundant Life Clinic has also conducted community HIV testing, counseled patients before and after testing, and offered prevention education.

Minority AIDS Project: Unity Fellowship Church, Los Angeles, California

Founded in 1985 by Bishop Carl Bean and the Unity Fellowship Church movement, the Minority AIDS Project (MAP) is the first community-based HIV/AIDS organization in the United States established and managed by people of color. The organization aims to make human services accessible to minorities in south central and central Los Angeles by designing culturally sensitive prevention education programs. MAP serves gay and bisexual men, women, the homeless, substance abusers, youth, ex-gang members, former inmates, and transsexuals. MAP's health education programs are responsible for at least 1,300 interventions a month. Among the organization's health education initiatives are early intervention, education, and treatment advocacy for people infected with HIV/AIDS; a behavior modification and maintenance program for substance abusers and the homeless; a needle exchange program; and a life skills and job training program for youth, former inmates, and ex-gang members. With a monthly caseload of 700, MAP's client services division provides case management, home health care, housing, and transportation assistance. It also operates mental health and support groups, a food pantry, clothing bank, and mobile testing unit. And a day program offers social and educational events, group bonding, case management, and psychological support to reduce the isolation that PWLAs often feel.

Sisters Together and Reaching (STAR): Baltimore, Maryland

STAR was founded in 1991 by Dorothy Brewster-Lee, MD, a family practitioner; Ernestine King-McCoy, a registered nurse; Debra Hickman, a clinical research nurse; and several other health care providers and Christian women. The organization aims to stem the spread of AIDS in the African-American community and to empower women to live in the midst of the AIDS epidemic with hope, awareness, and a regenerated spirit of wellness. STAR's staff, board members, and volunteers are all African-American women. This culturally sensitive environment helps build trust among clients.

STAR recruits and trains community volunteers to work one-on-one with women who are infected with AIDS. Through these pairings, Christian volunteers lend friendship and support to HIV-positive women. STAR also provides ongoing prevention education to the community, and gathers, sorts, and distributes information on HIV/AIDs-related issues. STAR coordinates many group activities, including workshops, peer education, weekly spiritual support group meetings, art therapy, and family gatherings that encourage familial support. The organization has also conducted several focus groups on the direct care needs of PWLAs in the Baltimore area. STAR provides emergency financial assistance for food, prescription medication, rent and utilities, and bus tokens.

The agency's community outreach efforts include a telephone helpline, health fairs, public forums, Street Outreach, and legislative updates. STAR also offers HIV/AIDS sensitivity training for churches, and helps churches and other community organizations to establish AIDS ministries.

Since its inception, STAR has served more than 700 women. In addition, the organization networks with other service providers in the city. As the organization's literature states, STAR provides "sisters with a comfortable place. . . where they can laugh, cry, share, and be themselves. They. . . will not be judged; but will get a big hug, a handful of tissues, and a compassionate listener who cares."

STAR has received funding from the Family Outreach Department of Total Health Care, Inc.; the Maryland State AIDS Administration; and the Baltimore Health Department. Grants have come from AIDSWALK, the St. Agnes Mission Fund, For Sisters Only, and individual donors. The organization has also been awarded contracts by the University of Maryland Medical System, Chase Brexton Health Services, and Johns Hopkins Women's Outreach.

Higher Dimensions: Tulsa, Oklahoma

In 1991 Higher Dimensions started SAFE (Serving AIDS-Impacted Families with Endurance) through its counseling center. The ministry, which lent support in a loving, accepting forum, aimed to help those affected by the virus better cope with the disease. The program components included a prayer support group; individual and group counseling; visitations to homebound shut-ins, hospitals, and prisons; and preventive education in schools, churches, housing projects, and community organizations. Twelve to fifteen people attended the weekly support group. SAFE also produced a biweekly radio program that was broadcast locally, and provided meals, transportation, housing locator assistance, and referrals to AIDS patients and their families.

"Our church got involved because we had members whose families were impacted by AIDS," counseling administrator Vanessa Vigers explained in a survey response. "God called forth laborers and we recognized the need to provide specialized ministry to those impacted."

The program ended in 1996 due to lack of volunteer support. However, the church continues to support efforts to minister to those infected and affected by HIV/AIDS. For example, the Higher Dimensions Asuza '97 Conference featured an address by Melody Crayton, the widow of an African-American minister who died of AIDS.

Trinity United Church of Christ: Chicago, Illinois

The AIDS ministry at Chicago's Trinity United Church of Christ started in 1992. According to Reverend Jeremiah Wright, pastor, the church's AIDS ministry addresses a full range of needs—from AIDS patients' initial diagnoses to their burials. "Our AIDS ministry volunteers have buried persons who are not members of this church whom they have met while working on the AIDS wards in the hospital," pastor Wright wrote in a December 1997 letter. "They have buried them, incidentally, using money out of their own pockets."

Teens, young adults, and other members of the church volunteer with the AIDS ministry that has served more than 200 people since its inception. The ministry is funded through the church's budget. In addition to providing pastoral care to PLWAs, the church has participated in worship services, seminars, workshops, and "teach-ins" in observance of World AIDS Day and African-American church AIDS Day. Further, Wright has preached several sermons on AIDS and homosexuality and has presided over numerous funerals of AIDS victims.

The pastor cites homophobia, denial, and lack of cooperation from other African-American churches as key challenges. He also complains that there are too few hospice facilities and insufficient funds for programs serving African-American PLWAs.

Friendship Ministries: Macon, Georgia

Reverend Sam Johnson, executive director of Friendship Ministries in Macon, Georgia, said he first encountered AIDS during his clinical training at Mercer Hospital. He later met a minister of music suffering from AIDS. The man died without ever disclosing that he had the disease or that he was gay. Johnson thought that the stigma that spurred such secrecy compounded physical suffering with loneliness.

His church took action when a social services agency called seeking assistance for an HIV/AIDS-infected mother and her four children. Friendship Ministries began as a shelter and housing development. The ministry, which stopped grouping the housing units together when they became labeled "an AIDS neighborhood," has housed 125 homeless families and provided temporary shelter for 1,800 nights.

The ministry not only offers assistance to the poor and disenfranchised but provides prevention education, as well. Friendship has initiated education projects for churches in thirteen rural counties and in several area schools.

Johnson said the ministry faces difficulty competing with white gay organizations for funds. The ministry is supported by the Georgia Department of Human Resources, the Georgia Department of Community Development, the congregation, and fund raisers.

Mt. Tabor Missionary Baptist Church: Miami, Florida

Pastored by George McCray, Mt. Tabor Missionary Baptist Church started MOVERS (Minorities Overcoming the Virus through Education, Responsibility, and Spirituality) in 1990. The AIDS ministry helps PLWAs obtain medication, medical assistance, housing, food, and counseling services, and conducts prevention education programs in local schools. The ministry has received funding from the Ryan White Fund, local government, and the United Methodist Board of Global Ministries' Health and Welfare Ministries Department. The church also allots 10 percent of its budget to outreach. Nevertheless, funding poses a constant challenge. "It is difficult to get funding diverted directly to the African-American community," Reverend McCray said in a February 1998 interview. "Some agencies don't understand that we can reach our people better than they can."

Glide/Goodlett AIDS Project:
San Francisco, California

With forty-two programs, Glide Memorial United Methodist Church is the largest private provider of social services in the San Francisco area. Reverend Cecil Williams, self-proclaimed minister of liberation since 1964, started preaching about AIDS in 1987, and organized church members to provide practical and emotional support to church members dealing with AIDS. Early on, the church sponsored a conference on AIDS for local clergy and caregivers.

In 1988, under the leadership of Williams and Reverend Louis Ashley, the church established the Glide/Goodlett AIDS Project—named for physician, newspaper publisher, and civil rights activist Carlton Goodlett. Acknowledging the link between drug abuse and unsafe sex, the ministry deems AIDS a recovery issue.

Like other Glide ministries, the AIDS project pursues a street outreach strategy. To reach at-risk groups, staff and volunteers approach people in parks, neighborhoods, and soup kitchen lines, distributing project information, bleach kits for IV drug users, and safer-sex kits, and offering free HIV testing at the church. The first church to offer HIV testing after worship service, Glide has tested 7,000 to 8,000 people over the years. In addition to testing, the church offers counseling, support groups, pastoral care, and prevention and support services. In January 1998, the project had a caseload of 300 to 400 clients. Further, a fifty-two-unit residential building for recovering addicts and individuals and families living with AIDS was under construction. The facility will be next door to the church. The majority of the AIDS ministry's funding comes from the San Francisco Department of Public Health.

Windsor Village United Methodist Church: Houston, Texas

Windsor's AIDS Ministry was founded in June 1989 to provide quality, culturally sensitive, and language-specific HIV/AIDS education and services to the black community. Incorporated in 1993 as the WAM Foundation, the ministry is located in a predominantly black section of southwest Houston. WAM provides education and social services, including professional counseling, case management, support groups, a speakers bureau, and financial assistance with rent, mortgage, and utility payments. Buddy teams link church volunteers with HIV/AIDS-infected clients or family members. Through visits and phone calls, buddies form one-on-one relationships, offering friendship and emotional support. Care teams provide support and physical care to HIV/AIDS patients and respite to their families. The food pantry distributes, and when necessary delivers, groceries to PLWAs on a biweekly basis. The outreach program locates high-risk populations in the community who are not linked with the HIV/AIDS Service System. And the teen posse uses teenage presenters to communicate prevention/education information to high-risk teens. The ministry has also sponsored back-to-school parties and has given out school supplies, clothes, holiday food baskets, and gifts. Under the leadership of pastor Kirbyjon Caldwell and executive director Brenda Smith, WAM annually provides educational services to 600 people and direct social services to 800 PLWAs. WAM cooperates with other HIV/AIDS service providers.

Ark of Refuge, Inc.: Oakland, California

Ark of Refuge grew out of a train-the-trainer peer outreach program cofounded by Reverend Yvette Flunder in 1988 to provide AIDS education to religious and lay communities. In 1989 the program expanded its scope to include housing and direct services for low-income and homeless PLWAs. The program created The Ark House, Oakland's first communal-living facility with comprehensive services. By 1991 the program had established a multi-denominational minister's Community Health Task Force, as well as the Women's Task Force on AIDS that trained church women as peer educators and group facilitators for programs targeting at-risk women and their children.

By 1992 the agency had been incorporated and granted nonprofit status. It had also administered a state-funded HIV education program serving clergy in San Francisco and Alameda Counties, and established the Hazard-Ashley House for homeless HIV-positive men. The ministry's housing programs now include Hazard-Ashley House; Walker House, which provides twenty-four-hour supportive care for end-stage and disabled AIDS/HIV patients with low or no income; and Restoration House, a dual-diagnosis facility with support and recovery services for African-American women. The agency provides case management services, individual counseling, needs assessment, and pastoral care.

The Ark also sponsors support groups and conducts workshops on HIV education, prevention, nutrition management, alternative treatments, and relapse prevention. Its peer education and prevention program has become a local and national model. In addition to targeting homosexuals and high-risk youth, the Ark also offers training for volunteers that lends practical and emotional support. The Ark shares its know-how through training manuals funded by the CDC and the Robert Woods Johnson Foundation.

The Ark's agenda, however, is not limited to training and housing programs; nor is it confined to East Oakland. The agency works with the Black Adoption Research and Placement Center to assist children orphaned by parents who succumbed to AIDS. The agency has also reached out to male and female inmates and to transgendered individuals with pastoral care, prevention education, and other services.

Under the leadership of cofounder Yvette Flunder, a gospel artist who pastors City of Refuge United Church of Christ, the Ark has targeted the gospel music industry and its fans. The agency developed CDC-funded outreach to the Gospel Music Workshop of America; worked with Baylor University; and The Balm in Gilead to enlist the support of the Gospel Music Announcers Association for the Black Church Week of Prayer for the Healing of AIDS. The Ark has also coproduced gospel music fund-raisers benefiting AIDS and each year presents an HIV-education workshop to the 40,000-member Gospel Music Workshop of America.

The organization also seeks to shape public policy, advocating for PLWAs in forums such as the National AIDS Roundtable, San Francisco Interreligious Coalition on AIDS, National African American Church Caucus on AIDS, and State of California Ryan White Working Group.

Goler Memorial A.M.E. Zion Church:
Winston-Salem, North Carolina

Reverend Seth Lartey, pastor of Goler Memorial A.M.E. Zion Church in Winston-Salem, North Carolina, believes that apathy is the greatest obstacle to the involvement of the African American church. Lartey's congregation, however, was moved to action when he delivered a sermon about a two-year-old and her mother, both of whom are infected with AIDS. They had no one to help them. After the sermon, Goler's members asked Lartey what they could do to help. They decided to adopt the mother and child. Members visited the family. Once they overcame the stigma associated with AIDS and realized the disease is not transmitted through casual contact, the church members began tending to the family's physical needs. As a safeguard, the AIDS ministry team received special training on handling and caring for babies and persons with AIDS.

In time, Goler's congregation witnessed the discrimination that some PLWAs experience. When the family's landlord discovered that the mother and daughter had AIDS, he threatened eviction. The church stepped in to advocate for the family. Had the members of the church not become directly involved, they might never have known how cruel society can be to PLWAs.

Goler's congregation continues to make small strides toward developing an AIDS ministry. Since adopting a family living with AIDS, the church has become interested in building a group home where AIDS patients can live and die in peace. One summer, the church devoted its Vacation Bible School to AIDS-prevention education.

Lartey contends, however, that the problems and needs of PLWAs are too great for one congregation to single-handedly address. He hopes that African-American churches in Winston-Salem will pool their resources to mount an effective ministry for people living with AIDS.

Chapter 9

In the Spirit of Cooperation

We don't need to reinvent the wheel. The church needs to partner with other organizations.[1]

Reverend Alfonso Wyatt

THE WISDOM OF PARTNERSHIPS

Some African-American pastors complain that their churches, and they themselves, are overburdened and overextended. African-American churches often lack the financial and human resources to implement outreach ministries. Given these constraints, mounting an AIDS ministry can be a daunting task.

"The most important thing that churches can do is to determine what it is they'd like to do," said theologian Wardell Payne in a January 1998 interview. "There are so many facets of serving people living with AIDS. Churches want to do everything, but they need to understand that they need to work in partnership with other congregations in their communities."

Miami minister George McCray agrees. "African-American churches should drop denominationalism to combat the AIDS problem," he said in a February 1998 interview.

In a funding environment that allegedly favors white gay AIDS organizations, partnerships are crucial to the effectiveness and survival of African-American AIDS ministries. The concept of partnerships not only involves African-American churches working together across denominations, but also with community organizations and established AIDS agencies to reach the underserved African-American community. In fact, more African-American churches probably support community-based AIDS efforts than operate independent AIDS ministries. Collaborative efforts range from prevention education and nutrition programs to case management. The following are a few of the partnerships forged by African-American churches.

MODEL PARTNERSHIPS

Allen Temple Baptist Church: Oakland, California

Allen Temple Baptist Church began its AIDS ministry in 1989 as the virus spread in the congregation. The ministry collaborates with Refuge Ministries HIV/AIDS program to provide case management services, food, and transportation to PLWAs. The project also provides housing assistance. It is working with the Allen Temple Housing and Economic Development Corporation to develop a supportive services plan for a twenty-four-unit housing project that the church is slated to construct for PLWAs. With a corps of volunteers consisting mainly of PLWAs and retirees, the ministry has served 150 to 200 clients. Volunteers visit PLWAs at home and in hospitals. Allen Temple's collaborative partner, Refuge Ministries, receives support from the Ryan White Fund.

God's Love We Deliver

God's Love We Deliver (GLWD) is a multimillion dollar, nonsectarian organization that prepares and delivers hot meals to homebound PLWAs in New York City and Hudson County, New Jersey. Founded in 1985, the agency began when Ganga Stone, a hospice volunteer, used an old bicycle to deliver meals donated by area restaurants. When demand increased, the operation moved from Stone's house into a church basement, then to a former nurse's home, and finally to Manhattan's trendy Soho neighborhood.

The agency operates through a network of more than sixty organizations and institutions known as neighborhood distribution centers. The centers accept delivery of insulated food tubs and oversee the distribution of food to clients via local volunteers. The volunteers not only deliver meals, but serve as oral historians for homebound PLWAs, taping their reminiscences for later transcription.

Three African-American churches serve as major distribution centers: Salem Missionary Baptist Church and Concord Baptist Church of Christ in Brooklyn; and Allen A.M.E. Church in Jamaica, Queens. Salem Missionary Baptist delivers 200 meals per week; Concord Baptist, 120; and Allen A.M.E., 250.

Allen covers the largest area in Queens and feeds the most clients. In addition, the parishioners who deliver meals use their own vehicles and incur their own gasoline expenses, which spares GLWD the usual delivery costs. In an August 1998 interview, Allen associate minister Alfonso Wyatt indicated that most of the church's volunteers are retirees. "These faithful volunteers have built a strong ministry of help as they reach out to deliver, not just food, but also concern, human contact, a smile, and precious words of encouragement," Wyatt said.

1997 Conference on HIV/AIDS and African Americans: Tulsa, Oklahoma

First Baptist Church of North Tulsa, a 500-member black congregation, spearheaded an April 1997 conference on HIV/AIDS. Presenting organizations included Love Center Christian Fellowship, Planned Parenthood of Tulsa, Rogers University, Tulsa Campus, and pharmaceutical companies. Event sponsors included the Indian Health Care Resource Center, Tulsa Area Chapter of the American Red Cross, Tulsa Association of Black Journalists, Regional AIDS Interfaith Network, Community of Hope United Methodist Congregation, Tulsa University, Higher Dimensions Family Church, and Revelations Revealed Truth Evangelistic Center. Among the event's supporters was the NAACP.

With a focus on prevention education, the conference targeted African Americans, teens, and young adults, and sought to bring the African-American community together in a spirit of solidarity and action against the AIDS epidemic. During the conference, youth played a *Jeopardy*-type game aimed at raising AIDS awareness; clergy participated in a roundtable discussion; and ministers and laypersons attended workshops on organizing AIDS ministries and creating partnerships between clergy, laity, and the community.

The Names Project Foundation

In ancient Africa and during the slavery era, textile arts such as quilting provided a utilitarian medium for expression. Through quilts, African descendants told their stories and preserved their memories. The AIDS Memorial Quilt serves a similar purpose. The quilt began with a square stitched by gay activist Cleve Jones in memory of his friend Marvin Feldman. The three-by-six-foot piece of cloth was a powerful symbol. Eventually, people from across the country began sending quilt panels to the San Francisco storefront that housed what had become known as the Names Project. In October 1997, volunteers unfurled 2,000 quilt panels on the National Mall in Washington, DC. The solemn ritual and heart-rending display opened hearts and minds to the reality that everyone is affected by AIDS.

The quilt now contains more than 40,000 panels adorned with photographs, mementos, prayers, and messages by tens of thousands of people from around the globe. Represented in the massive quilt are panels crafted by families or friends of numerous African-American AIDS victims. Each year, the Names Project and its forty-one chapters sponsor nearly 1,800 displays nationwide in schools, offices, hospitals, shopping malls, community centers, and places of worship where they are seen by nearly 2.5 million people.

The National Interfaith Quilt Program allows churches and religious groups to display small portions of the AIDS Memorial Quilt for a period of up to one month. Participating faith communities also receive a program handbook; public relations, media, and education kits; a video presentation; and technical assistance. The Quilt Program offers solace to the bereaved, support for PLWAs, inclusion for the marginalized, and hope in the face of despair. Several African-American churches have participated in the Quilt Program, including St. George Episcopal Church in Brooklyn, New York; Calvary Temple Baptist Church in Kansas City, Missouri; and Memorial Baptist Church in New York City. In 1997, historically black North Carolina A&T State University displayed the quilt on its Greensboro campus.

Chapter 10

Africa: From Cradle to Grave

He who recognizes the disease is the physician.

African proverb

EPICENTER OF THE GLOBAL EPIDEMIC

AIDS is devastating Africa. In Uganda the AIDS epidemic has created a brisk market for coffins. In one village, coffin manufacturing is a cottage industry. Some workers plane wood, while older children help stack handmade coffins in a small shack. The AIDS epidemic assures there will be a steady stream of bereaved customers. These coffins will ensure that the dead have decent burials.

More than two-thirds of all adults living with HIV/AIDS live in sub-Saharan Africa. By July 1996, the region had lost more than three million people to AIDS. And a November 1997 World Bank report indicated that fourteen million people in sub-Saharan Africa were HIV positive—the world's highest rate of infection.[1] The United Nations Program on AIDS (UNAIDS) estimates that half of the adult population in some cities in Zambia, Malawi, and Botswana are HIV positive. South African health officials report that 1,500 South Africans are infected with the virus every day, and project that as many as two million South Africans could be unaware they are infected.

In 1987 President Kenneth Kaunda of Zambia disclosed that his son, Masuzga, who died in 1986, had AIDS. The first African leader to announce that a member of his family had AIDS, Kaunda called for an African offensive on the disease.

A decade later, Nigeria's most famous pop star, Fela Anikulapo-Kuti, died of the disease. His death in August 1997 made AIDS a hot topic in that country. Later that year, Judith Attah, the country's minister of women's affairs and social welfare, reported that 2.25 million Nigerians are infected. "It will not be too long before we share the plight of some countries where entire adult populations of men and women in the villages are virtually wiped out by the AIDS scourge, leaving behind only children," Attah warned.[2]

AIDS not only affects the health of African people, but also national economies. The World Bank projects that in the year 2010, Tanzania's economy will be a quarter less than it would have been without AIDS.[3] AIDS is also financially taxing for families living with the disease. Loss of income combined with health care costs reduce the funds available for home care, an option preferred by most African PLWAs.

At a December 1997 meeting of the Zimbabwean conference of the United Methodist Church, Bishop Christopher Jokomo lamented, "AIDS is becoming a disease of poor people."

AFRICAN FACES OF AIDS

Heterosexual transmission predominates in sub-Saharan Africa. Women and children are most at risk for infection. According to UNAIDS, more than six million women of childbearing age are infected. As many as one million children may have been infected during pregnancy, delivery, or breast-feeding.[4] The number of women infected outnumbers men six to five. In Uganda, five times as many young women aged fifteen to nineteen are infected as young men of the same age.[5]

Several factors have contributed to the rapid spread of AIDS in the region: population movements spurred by conflict, famine or poverty; the prevalence of other sexually transmitted diseases that, if left untreated, increase the AIDS risk; and the lower status of women. Biologically, epidemiologically, and socially, women are more vulnerable to infection. Women tend to marry older men, who have had multiple sexual partners and are more likely to be infected. In some cultures it is virtually impossible for women to insist that their husbands be monogamous or use condoms. Further, men in some societies demand and expect sex from any women receiving their financial support. Such cultural and religious inhibitions have hampered prevention efforts in Africa.

In December 1992, the Seventh International Conference on AIDS in Africa convened in Yaounde, Cameroon. At the time, pharmaceutical treatment for AIDS was almost nonexistent in Africa. Sy Al Hadj Amadou, then African Secretary of the International Council of AIDS Service Organizations, said the continent's anti-AIDS efforts had been rendered ineffective by the lack of access to AIDS treatments. In the absence of treatment options, prevention tactics cannot reaffirm life or promise hope. Consequently, prevention education loses credibility. These issues, said Amadou, have created a climate of neglect.

Noticeably absent from the conference were the traditional medical practitioners who are many Africans' first line of defense against illness. Though largely ignored by Western-oriented development agencies, these healers, regarded as physicians and priests, are a vital part of the African health care system. With their ties to the people, traditional healers could play a crucial role in education, prevention, and treatment.

Fokoundang Adam Usumanu, the one traditional healer who attended the conference, planned to organize traditional medical practitioners in Cameroon to pool their knowledge and resources to help treat AIDS patients. Usumanu has had some success in using yohimbine bark to treat fatigue in AIDS patients.

Still, pharmaceutical treatments are sorely needed in Africa. During the conference, Jonathan Mann, a professor at Harvard School of Public Health, announced the creation of a new center at Harvard University for the study of health and human rights. He observed that people who have their rights generally have their health as well.

Human rights and medical ethics are central to the debate surrounding sixteen studies being sponsored by the the CDC and National Institutes of Health in developing countries. The studies seek cheap and practical alternatives to AZT, a treatment proven effective in preventing the spread of AIDS from mother to child. At a treatment cost of $1,000 per pregnant woman, AZT is too pricey for women in Africa, where per capita spending on health care is less than $10 a year.

In U.S. studies, participants in all comparison groups are given a longer regimen of AZT. In these cost-cutting third world studies, however, the pregnant, HIV-positive women received a brief regimen of AZT or no treatment at all. Allegedly, some of the poor, mostly uneducated women did not understand that they might get a placebo or that AZT was already known to prevent the transmission of the virus during pregnancy. Such tests would be illegal in the United States. *The New England Journal of Medicine* compared these clinical trials to the infamous Tuskegee Syphilis Study.

In October 1997, Bernice Powell Jackson, executive director of the United Church of Christ's Commission for Racial Justice, exposed the study in "Civil Rights Journal." The editorial column, which appears in many African-American newspapers, posed troubling questions about the government tests using the poor and people of color. "What is the ethics of only the rich of the world having access to life-saving drugs?" Jackson asked.[6]

A NEW AFRICAN MISSION

While the pharmaceutical industry and medical community ponder ethical questions, AIDS is claiming the lives of more and more young Africans each week. During the June 1993 International HIV/AIDS Conference in Berlin, Germany, an HIV-positive participant from Zimbabwe charged that organized religion is "guilty of comfortable compassion."[7]

Similarly, a 1996 report by the World Council of Churches (WCC) said that, for the most part, churches' response to AIDS "has been inadequate and has, in some cases made the problem worse." The report charged that "many Christians and some churches shared in the promotion of negative judgmental and condemnatory attitudes." The WCC challenged churches to side-step their theological and ethical differences about sexuality to fight AIDS.[8]

In Kenya, for example, two denominations opposed a government-sponsored family life education program that covered contraception and condom use. In August 1995, Roman Catholic Cardinal Maurice Otunga and Muslim leader Ali Shee staged a public protest against the sex education program. The two clergymen burned sex education literature and condoms in Nairobi's Uhuru Park.

In Africa, denominational views sometimes clash with cultural traditions as well. African spirituality is rooted in history, culture, family, and custom. In traditional African culture, man's physical needs and spiritual nature are intertwined, and religion is deemed a healing force. Through colonialism and Christian missions, the church gained vast influence in many parts of Africa. In some countries, the first schools, hospitals, and clinics were church affiliated. The contemporary African church is ideally suited to mount grassroots programs and educate the masses.

Traditional African values, however, have hampered AIDS education and prevention efforts, said Dr. Musimbi Kanyoro, a Kenyan who heads the Lutheran World Federation's office on women in society. During a November 1997 meeting of the Lutheran AIDS Network, she explained, "Many Africans maintain that the African traditional morality ensured the integrity of the society and individuals." This abandonment of old cultural practices has wrought social and psychological disorder.

Kanyoro said African morality held "that spiritual powers are deeply concerned about the moral conduct of individuals and communities alike. There are many for whom this disease is nothing other than God's punishment for evils done by society." Such beliefs, she contended, obscure the scientific facts of transmission and treatment. "Although the link between AIDS and sexual behavior is now scientifically well-established, in many parts of Africa a change in sexual behavior does not follow."

Kanyoro stressed that AIDS educators focus on oral communication in rural areas to compensate for high illiteracy and a lack of electricity for radio and television.

In 1987, the Methodist Church in Kenya took initiative by piloting a program that prepared parents to teach responsible sexual behavior to their children. During the early 1990s, most religious groups in Kenya either ignored the AIDS crisis or blamed the epidemic on immorality. Churches shunned PLWAs until they became gravely ill, and some clergy even led anticondom campaigns, fearing prevention education would encourage promiscuity.

Meanwhile, a less vocal group of clergy sought interventions. Those religious leaders formed the nucleus of the MAP Kenya HIV/AIDS Project. MAP, a nondenominational, nonprofit, Christian relief and development organization, had already been working on health care and community development with churches, government agencies, and other institutions. When MAP shared with Kenyan clergy that 49 percent of young churchgoers had premarital sex, the ministers were compelled to act. They were also shocked that so many Kenyans held misconceptions about the epidemic.

To better equip pastors to address these issues, MAP provides training in pastoral counseling; counseling, social service, and prevention education manuals; curriculum modules; and awareness packets with posters, brochures, a Bible study text, and scripturally based AIDS sermon outlines. MAP also publishes a guide to help parents bridge the communication gap to educate their children about sex. The guide helps fill the void left by increased urbanization, the decline of the extended family, and rites of passage which traditionally taught children about sex.

In 1994 the Kenyan Christian AIDS Network grew out of MAP's efforts to unite various Kenyan denominations on policy issues. In November 1994 Kenyan religious leaders met and adopted a general position statement on HIV/AIDS. The succinct statement committed churches to "a ministry of Christian hope, reconciliation, and healing in our congregations and communities through prevention, education, and care for persons and families."[9]

We have mentioned but a few of Africa's church-based AIDS initiatives. In Mombasa, Kenya, the Church of the Province of Kenya employed proverbs to convey sex education messages. Several African proverbs seem appropriate for the AIDS pandemic:

Instruction in youth is like engraving in stones.

That which is deadly may have a sweet scent.

What happens to your wife happens to yourself.

The stick that is to save you is found in your hand.

When cows are about to go out, they lick one another; when men are about to die they love one another.

An African-American church mother might add these words of wisdom: "Where there's a will there's a way."

The African church has demonstrated that it has the will to fight AIDS, despite dire poverty that limits treatment options, dashes hope, and dooms PLWAs to die.

During the Ninth International Congress on HIV/AIDS that convened in June 1993 in Berlin, Episcopal Bishop Kauma of Uganda said he valued the experience of ministering to PLWAs. "The church in Uganda," he attested, "has been brought closer to God through working with persons infected with HIV."[10]

Creationists and anthropologists alike consider Africa the cradle of civilization. In the absence of proven AIDS treatments, though, the continent could well become the graveyard of humanity.

Chapter 11

A Sense of Loss, a Sense of Purpose

AIDS is the most devastating pandemic that modern man has encountered. The epidemic hit home for us (the authors), not when the media reported alarming infection and morbidity rates, but when the disease struck those we loved. Ron has lost three cousins and several friends to AIDS. He shares his experiences here.

FAMILY FUNERALS

My cousin Derek, whom I once baby-sat, was diagnosed with AIDS after returning from Florida, where he had fled as a runaway. I had not seen him for several years when we renewed our ties at a family reunion. I told him I had entered the ministry. He indicated that he was gay and HIV positive, but he had made peace with God and his fate. A year later, I heard he was in the end stages of the disease. When I phoned I found that Derek had healed his relationship with his father, who had become his caretaker.

My cousin Debbie contracted AIDS from her husband, an IV drug user. She was very angry and she was concerned about what would happen to her three children upon her death. When she died, her aunt cared for her youngest child.

My cousin Leroy, an accomplished vocalist, lived in New York. The last time I saw him was when he sang at my brother's wedding. When he became ill, he moved in with his mother, who had returned to the small town where she had grown up. He died in her care.

FRIENDS FOR LIFE

My friend Jason died in 1995. In the neighborhood where I grew up, he was one of the older guys everyone looked up to. Generous to a fault, Jason shared everything he had, opening his home to friends day in and day out. On a visit home, I passed him on the street and he did not recognize me. His complexion was blotched and he had lost a lot of weight. Since he used intravenous drugs, I immediately suspected that he had AIDS. My brother confirmed that such a rumor had been circulating. A few months later, Jason was dead.

The AIDS death that hit me hardest, however, was that of my boyhood friend Tony. We were like brothers, getting into all kinds of mischief together. When I visited home as an adult, he was the only friend I could count on seeing. Tony had a secret side, however, that I discovered when I once dropped by his house unannounced. His mother told me that he had stolen and pawned his sister's stereo system, and asked me to drive her to get it out of hock. This provoked me to confront Tony about rumors of his drug use. I never gave up on our friendship and continually urged him to kick his heroin and cocaine habit. In time, he got clean, landed a job as bail bondsman, and fell in love with the woman who would become his third wife. A premarital blood test revealed that he was HIV positive. Depressed, he phoned and told me he was infected. Unsure whether he had contracted AIDS by having sex with prostitutes or using dirty needles, Tony swore me to secrecy, fearing he would become a social outcast. Besides being bitter, he worried he had infected his fiancée and wondered whether they should still marry. She was HIV negative; they married, but separated after a couple of years.

A father of four, Tony moved into his mother's home. I visited him several times there. He believed that God had forgiven him and confessed that he needed God in his life. But he feared he would be rejected by the Episcopal parish in which he was baptized as a boy. Nevertheless, he renewed his ties to his family's church. Some parishioners spread rumors that he was homosexual, and the church offered him little support beyond pastoral visits. In fact, a somewhat judgmental minister almost alienated him.

Despite the church's response, Tony's faith deepened as his body weakened. He believed God would heal him and denied that he was going to die. During his most serious health crisis, this faith may have helped him cope with the possibility of death. Sometimes when I called, he was too weak to lift the phone to his ear; his mother conveyed messages between us.

On my last visit, Tony expressed regret about his lifestyle choices. He desperately hoped his children would never get AIDS. As my friend lay dying he urged me to use the pulpit to help people understand that AIDS can be prevented by avoiding risky behavior. "Tell people to live right," he ordered. I knew I would never again see him alive. We embraced. I thanked him for his friendship, and he assured me that we would see each other again someday. At that moment, I realized the true meaning of healing.

There is a difference between a healing and cure. Healing occurs when broken family relations are mended and family members accept each other unconditionally. Healing occurs when a person's self-image is restored and when the burden of guilt is lifted. Healing occurs when people like Tony have faith in God's promise of everlasting life. By becoming the hands of God, the church can offer PLWAs this assurance.

CRUSADE AGAINST AIDS

Now more than ever, African-American clergy must practice what they preach. Here, then is "The African American Clergy's Declaration of War on HIV/AIDS." Adopted during the 1994 African-American Religious Leaders Summit on HIV/AIDS at the White House, it offers a potent prescription for AIDS intervention and prevention:

> The time has come today to face the depth of devastation caused by AIDS in the African-American community; to recognize that African Americans are the most disproportionately represented community of color with respect to HIV/AIDS; that AIDS continues to be the leading cause of death nationwide of African-American men between 35 and 44, and of African-American women between the ages of 25 and 44; that the number of teenagers infected with HIV doubles each year; and that each and every American knows someone, or in the next 12 months will know someone who has died of AIDS.
>
> The African-American Church has a long and distinguished tradition of leading its people to light in times of great suffering, and of caring for its parishioners. It has a proud history of pastoral activism and has proven itself a formidable mobilizer of congregations. But the time has come today to recognize that as far as our churches have come in the night, there are steps yet to go before dawn; that the African-American religious community, despite this legacy, has too long been negligent on the pressing subject of HIV/AIDS. The church's godly mission is to minister love and support to its congregations, and to forsake no one. Yet, until today, it has not assumed its proper mantle of responsibility in this time of chaos caused by the ravages of AIDS to mind, body, and soul of our people.
>
> Now, therefore, we, leaders of African-American churches in America, deem it necessary to acknowledge by means of this proclamation that only through stalwart commitment, strength of mind, and courage of heart on the part of the religious community, can we ever hope to combat the AIDS epidemic. By this proclamation, we declare our intent to do

all in our power to eradicate the scourge of AIDS in our time; to wage war on fear and ignorance of AIDS/HIV, from the pulpit and in our institutions, until such time that AIDS is no longer a threat to the lives of the people, and we call upon our fellow clergy, men and women, to do the same.

We, members of the clergy of African-American churches in America, recognize that as long as one human being remains uneducated, as long as one human being suffers from AIDS, it is one too many; we vow to develop comprehensive AIDS prevention programs for our youth; to develop effective AIDS awareness and prevention strategies for and with our congregations and communities; to provide supportive counseling to Persons Living with AIDS and to their noninfected families and loved ones; and to preach consciousness-raising sermons about AIDS prevention and compassion for all, regardless of sexual orientation, drug dependency, or lifestyle choices.

We furthermore affirm our commitment to working with grassroots organizations, corporations, and governmental bodies on the federal, state, and municipal levels to secure generous financial support of AIDS awareness and prevention and to educate our congregations in those programs; and to work throughout our own institutions, the seminaries and schools of theology, to combat silence on the subject of AIDS and promote an enlightened, nonjudgmental clergy, unimpeded in the war on AIDS by nonproductive biases.

We furthermore affirm our commitment to identifying tangible goals and means of assessing progress on these goals, formulating policy, and engaging in advocacy on behalf of our communities with respect to the issues around AIDS.

We furthermore affirm our support for The Black Church National Day of Prayer for the Healing of AIDS as a vehicle for mobilizing African-American religious institutions to fight AIDS through prayer, education, and advocacy nation-wide. And in this resolve advocate for universal health care.

We furthermore affirm that from this day forward, we resolve to open our eyes and acknowledge those persons among us living with AIDS and their families and loved ones, and to encourage others to see; to open our ears to their voices among us, and to insist that others hear; to open our hearts in compassion, and expect others to do the same, and in so doing, cast off the denial that has hindered our churches in the past, and in so doing move forward with a sense of divine mission to educate our communities, our congregations and our fellow clergy about AIDS, and in so doing, say at last,

Surely, there is a balm in Gilead.[1]

Pray that this activist rhetoric breathes life into AIDS ministries and saves lives in the African-American community.

Appendix A

Why the African-American Church Must Liberate the Community from AIDS

These statements are not necessarily listed in order of importance.

1. AIDS is not a quality-of-life issue; it's a life-or-death issue.
2. AIDS is spreading more rapidly in the African-American community. African Americans are six times more likely than whites to be infected with HIV/AIDS.
3. Although representing only 13 percent of the U.S. population, in 1996 African Americans represented a larger proportion (41 percent) of newly reported AIDS cases than whites (38 percent).
4. History has shown that the African-American pulpit has the power to educate, influence, and mobilize the masses.
5. The church has a responsibility to teach values and change behavior. For generations, the African-American church has been an arbiter of social norms.
6. The church is called to relieve suffering and offer hope.
7. The church was commissioned to minister to poor, sick, ignorant, marginalized, and underserved people.
8. As the hands of God, the church must not only save souls but save lives.
9. AIDS is the most serious crisis facing descendants of Africa since the slave trade.

10. If the rapid spread of AIDS continues, the African-American community will share the plight of some African nations where entire generations have been wiped out, leaving behind only children and the elderly.

Appendix B

First Steps to Forming AIDS Ministries

1. Determine the congregation's attitudes about AIDS.
2. Determine local needs and existing services by contacting area AIDS ministries, AIDS advocacy groups, and health agencies.
3. Invite people living with AIDS to share their stories with the congregation.
4. Conduct AIDS education for church leaders.
5. Determine the congregation's commitment and capacity to volunteer.
6. Define the ministry's focus: spiritual nurture, support, child care, housing, financial aid, fund-raising, Street Outreach, advocacy, pastoral care, and/or prevention education.
7. Determine whom the ministry will serve: people living with AIDS, at-risk populations, youth, women, older adults, etc.
8. Consider partnering with other congregations, AIDS organizations or health agencies.
9. Seek technical assistance from experienced AIDS program specialists.
10. Set a budget for the ministry.

Appendix C

Major Obstacles to Involvement

These obstacles are not necessarily listed in order of importance.

1. Perception that AIDS is punishment for sin
2. Myths about AIDS transmission
3. Conspiracy theories/Tuskegee Syphillis Study
4. Homophobia
5. Stigma linked to intravenous drug use
6. Reluctance to discuss sexuality
7. Reluctance to promote condom use
8. Fear of facing death
9. Lack of volunteers
10. Lack of funds

Appendix D

Directory of AIDS Resources

AIDS National Interfaith Network
1400 I Street, NW
Suite 1220
Washington, DC 20005
phone: (202) 842-0010
fax: (202) 842-3323
web site: www.thebody.com

Ark of Refuge
432 Mason Street
San Francisco, CA 94102
phone: (415) 778-1241

The Balm in Gilead
130 West 42nd Street
Suite 450
New York, NY 10036
phone: (212) 730-7381
fax: (212) 730-2551

Centers for Disease Control and Prevention (CDC)
Faith Initiative
1600 Clifton Road, NE
Mail Stop E-58
Atlanta, GA 30333
phone: (404) 639-5224
fax: (404) 639-5258

Congress of National Black Churches
1225 I Street, NW
Suite 750
Washington, DC 20005-3914
phone: (202) 371-1091
fax: (202) 371-0908

Leading for Life Campaign
Harvard AIDS Institute
651 Huntington Avenue
Boston, MA 02115
phone: (617) 432-4400
fax: (617) 432-4545
web site:
    www. hsph.harvard.edu/Organizations/hai/leading/leading.html

National AIDS Clearinghouse
P.O. Box 6003
Rockville, MD 20849-6003
phone: 1-800-458-5231
fax: (301) 738-6616

National Medical Association
1012 10th Street, NW
Washington, DC 20001
phone: (202) 347-1895
fax: (202) 842-3293

National Minority AIDS Council
1931 13th Street, NW
Washington, DC 20009-4432
phone: (202) 483-6622
fax: (202) 438-1135

Notes

Chapter 1

1. Leroy Whitfield, "Black plague," *Positively Aware*, (September/October 1997), Vol. 8, No. 5, 46.
2. Lloyd Gite, "The new agenda of the black church: Economic development for black America," (December 1993), *Black Enterprise*, 56.
3. Jerry M. Guess, "Freedom's warriors: The fighting black clergy, a historical view," (June/July 1990), *Crisis*, 30.
4. Pernessa Seele, founder and director, The Balm in Gilead, New York, NY, (February 11, 1998), phone interview by authors.
5. Al Sharpton, Brooklyn, NY, (February 6, 1998), phone interview by authors.
6. Seele, Ibid.
7. Andres Tapia, "Soul searching: How is the black church responding to the urban crisis?" *Christianity Today*, (March 1996), reprinted in Harambee Archives, http://www.harambee.org/archive/soul.html, 9.
8. Arthur Ashe and Arnold Rampersad, *Days of Grace*, (Thorndike, ME: G.K. Hall and Co., 1993), 205.
9. Mario Cooper, "The AIDS crisis within the African-American community," *Themis*, (Vol. 1, Issue 1, October/November 1997), http://www.iapac.org/minorities/themis.html), 6.
10. The Harvard AIDS Institute. "The AIDS crisis among African Americans: A report from the first leading for life summit," (October 22, 1996), 4.
11. Carlton Veazey, letter of welcome, "National black religious summit on sexuality: Breaking the silence," (May 7, 1997), Religious Coalition for Reproductive Choice, 3.
12. Carlton Veazey, executive director, Religious Coalition for Reproductive Choice, (January 25, 1998), phone interview by authors.
13. The Associated Press, "Black ministers say their churches should battle AIDS," (March 1, 1997), *Baltimore Afro-American*, A-12.
14. C. Eric Lincoln, *The Black Experience in Religion*, (Garden City, NY: Anchor/Doubleday, 1974), 55.

Chapter 2

1. The Harvard AIDS Institute. "The AIDS crisis among African Americans: A report from the first leading for life summit," (October 22, 1996), 3.

2. The screening of donated blood has greatly reduced the likelihood of the transfusion of tainted blood.

3. Unless otherwise noted all statistics come from the U.S. Department of Health and Human Services, Centers for Disease Control and Prevention.

4. Hanna Rosin, "The homecoming," (June 5, 1995), *The New Republic*, 22.

5. Alexandra Greeley, "Concern about AIDS in minority communities," (December 1995), *FDA Consumer,* http://www.fda.gov/fdac/features/095_aids.html, 3.

6. Abdul Alim Muhammad, MD, "HIV/AIDS in the African-American community," Nation of Islam Ministry of Health and Human Services, (July 29, 1997), http://www.noihealth.org/hivedu.html, 1.

7. The Harvard AIDS Institute, "The AIDS crisis among African Americans: A report from the first leading for life summit," (October 22, 1996), 3.

8. Otis Tillman, MD, *A Prescription for the Soul: Prayers and Meditations,* (High Point, NC: The Marshall Group, 1995), 12.

9. Ibid., 13.

Chapter 3

1. Laura Meckler, "AIDS compared to civil rights fight," (July 29, 1998), The Associated Press, 1-2.

2. Robert Thomas, "Heaven's bleach will kill your AIDS virus," *Nashville Pride*, (October 18, 1997), 4.

3. Pernessa Seele, founder and director, The Balm in Gilead, New York, NY, (February 11, 1998), phone interview by authors.

4. Gregory M. Herek and John Capitanio, "AIDS stigma and contact with persons with AIDS: Effects of direct and vicarious contact," *Journal of Applied Social Psychology,* Vol. 27 No. 1, (1997): 1-36.

5. Gregory M. Herek and John Capitanio, "Public reaction to AIDS in the United States: A second decade of stigma," *American Journal of Public Health*, (Vol. 83, No. 4, April 1993), 576.

6. Herek and Capitanio, *Journal of Applied Social Psychology,* Vol. 27 No. 1, (1997) 27.

7. Seth C. Kalichman, "Magic Johnson and public attitudes toward AIDS: A review of empirical findings," *AIDS Education and Prevention* (Vol. 6, No. 6, 1994), 545; citing A.A. Gleghorn, J.B. Jemmott, D. D. Celentano, and K.M. Kilbourn, "Magic Johnson's HIV Status: Impact on African-American STD patients." Paper presented at American Psychological Association, Toronto, Canada, August 1993.

8. Herek and Capitanio, *Journal of Applied Social Psychology* Vol. 27 No. 1, (1997) 5: citing T.L. Hunter, S.C. Kalichman, R.L. Russell, and D.B. Sarwer, "Earvin 'Magic' Johnson's HIV serostatus disclosure: Effects on men's perceptions of AIDS," *Journal of Consulting and Clinical Psychology*, Vol. 61, 887-891.

9. Keith Boykin, *One More River to Cross: Black and Gay in America,* (New York: Doubleday, 1996), 121-122.

10. "AIDS issue fades among Americans," *The Gallup Poll: Public Releases from Gallup Poll Results*, (1997), www.gallup.com/poll/news/971017.html.

11. Andrew M. Greeley, "Religion and attitudes toward AIDS policy." In Kenneth R. Overberg, *AIDS, Ethics and Religion: Embracing a World of Suffering*, (Maryknoll, NY: Orbis Books, 1994): 223-224.

12. "Americans worry over AIDS," *Reuters*, (December 4, 1997), http://204. 202.137. 113/sections/living/aidssurvey1204/index.html.

13. Harriet Washington, "HIV Among African Americans," *Harvard AIDS Review*, Spring/Summer 1996, http://www.hsph.harvard.edu/Organizations/haiini/publicat/review/sprsum_96.html, 6.

14. Sara Rimer, "Blacks urged to increase awareness of AIDS epidemic," *New York Times News Service*, (October 23, 1996), 1-2, http://plato.divanet.com/mansco/qnn/1996/hv6oct/HV207003.TXT.

15. Al Sharpton, Brooklyn, NY, (February 6, 1998), phone interview by authors.

16. Kenya Briggs, "A Look at Conflict and Opportunities for Dialogue Between African American and Lesbian/Gay/Bisexual Communities," *Crossroads*, (February 1994), America Online.

17. Alexandra Greeley, "Concern about AIDS in minority communities," (December 1995), *FDA Consumer*, http://www.fda.gov/fdac/features/095_aids.html, 4.

18. Hanna Rosin, "The homecoming," (June 5, 1995), *The New Republic*, 23.

19. Jeff Stryker, "Tuskegee's long arm still touches a nerve," (April 13, 1997), *The New York Times*, http://www.drugfreeamerica.org/inhale_ne.html, 1-3.

20. *The Chronicle* (Winston-Salem, NC), "Apology paves way," May 22, 1997, 12.

21. Boykin, 126.

22. Rhonda Graham, "And the choir sings on," *Wilmington News Journal*, October 23, 1994, America Online.

23. Ibid.

24. Ibid.

Chapter 4

1. James Cone, *A Black Theology of Liberation: Twentieth Anniversary Edition*, (Maryknoll, NY: Orbis Books, 1990), 11.

2. Letty Russell, ed., *The Church with AIDS*, (Louisville, KY: Westminister/ John Knox Press, 1990), 40: citing Kevin Gordon, "The sexual bankruptcy of Christian traditions: A perspective of radical suspicion and fundamental trust," David G. Halliman, ed., *AIDS Issues: Confronting the Challenge*, (New York: Pilgrim Press, 1989), 197-198.

3. Pernessa Seele, founder and director, The Balm in Gilead, New York, NY, (February 11, 1998), phone interview by authors.

4. Cecil Williams with Rebecca Lard, *No Hiding Place: Empowerment and Recovery for Our Troubled Communities*, (San Francisco, CA: Harper Collins Publishers, 1992), 216.

5. Carlton Veazey, executive director, Religious Coalition for Reproductive Choice, (January 25, 1998), phone interview by authors.

6. Yvette Flunder, "No doors on our huts: Celebrating community on the margin," master's thesis, Pacific School of Religion, www.sfrefuge.org/thesis/thesis2.html,3.

7. Alfonso Delany, pastor, Ebenezer United Methodist Church, Miami, FL, (February 2, 1998), phone interview by authors.

8. Daniel L. Migliore, *Faith Seeking Understanding: An Introduction to Christian Theology,* (Grand Rapids, MI: W.M.B. Eerdmans Publishing Company, 1991), 104-106.

9. Carlyle Fielding Stewart, III. *African-American Church Growth: 12 Principles for Prophetic Ministry* (Nashville, TN: Abington Press, 1994), 95.

10. Flunder, 2.

11. "African-American church summit breaks the silence on sexuality," *Religious Coalition for Reproductive Choice,* (Summer 1997), 3.

Chapter 5

1. Harriet Washington, "HIV Among African Americans," *Harvard AIDS Review,* (Spring/Summer 1996), www.hsph.harvard.edu/Organizations/hai.

2. Kenneth Miller, "A Church for the Twenty-First Century," *Life,* (April 1997), 50.

3. *The black church week of prayer for the healing of AIDS,* (1997). The Balm in Gilead, New York, 6.

Chapter 6

1. "African-American church summit breaks the silence on sexuality," *Religious Center for Reproductive Choice News,* (Summer 1997), pp.2-3.

2. Wardell Payne, (January 19, 1998), phone interview by authors.

3. Howard C. Stevenson Jr., "The psychology of sexual racism and AIDS: An ongoing saga of distrust and the 'sexual other,'" *Journal of Black Studies,* (Vol. 25, No. 1, September 1994), 62-80.

4. Mariah Britton, "Breaking silence," *Yes! Journal of Positive Futures*, Winter 1997/1998, 31.

5. Michael Eric Dyson, *Race Rules,* (New York: Addison-Wesley Publishing Company, 1996), 94.

Chapter 7

1. Beverly Hall Lawrence, *Reviving the Spirit,* (New York: Grove Press, 1996), 58.

2. C. Eric Lincoln and Lawrence H. Mamiya, *The Black Church in the African-American Experience,* (Durham, NC: Duke University Press, 1990): 128-131.

3. Don Nations, "10 assurances of pastoral care for those infected or affected by HIV/AIDS," *HIV/AIDS Ministries Network Focus Paper #22,* (New York: No-

vember 1993), Health and Welfare Program Ministries Program Department, General Board of Global Ministries, The United Methodist Church, 5.

4. Carolyn McCrary, "Interdependence as a normative value in pastoral counseling with African Americans," *The Journal of the I.T.C.*, (Vol. XVIII, Nos. 1 and 2, Fall/Spring 1990/1991), 143.

5. Edward P. Wimberly, "Pastoral counseling with African-American males," *The Journal of the I.T.C.*, (Vol. XXI, Nos. 1 and 2, Fall/Spring 1993/1994), 127-144.

Chapter 8

1. "Joycelyn Elders," Debra Gilliam Straub (ed.), *Voices of Multicultural America*, (Detroit: Gale Research, 1996): 359.

2. Centers for Disease Control and Prevention, "CDC HIV Prevention Faith Initiative," 1998.

3. Mary R. Sawyer, *Black Ecumenism: Implementing the Demands of Justice*, (Valley Forge, PA: Trinity Press International, 1994), 62.

4. Ibid., pp. 168-170.

5. The Balm in Gilead, "The black church week of prayer for the healing of AIDS," (New York: The Balm in Gilead, 1997).

6. The Balm in Gilead, Inc., "The African American clergy's declaration of war on HIV/AIDS," Resolution adopted at the First African American Religious Leaders Summit on HIV/AIDS, Washington, DC, February 28, 1995.

7. Abdul Alim Muhammad, MD, "HIV/AIDS in the African-American community," Nation of Islam Ministry of Health and Human Services, (July 29, 1997), http://www.noihealth.org/hivedu.html, 1-2; http://www.noihealth.org/hivtest.html, 1-2; http://www.noihealth.org/hivedu.html, 1-2; http://www.noihealth.org/hivcoun.html, 1; http://www.noihealth.org/hivtrem.html, 1-2; http://www.noihealth.org/hivres.html, 1-2; http://www.noihealth.org/hivinf.html, 1-2; http://www.noihealth.org/hivglob.html, 1-2;

Chapter 9

1. Reverend Alfonso Wyatt, associate pastor, Allen A.M.E. Church, Jamaica, NY, August 13, 1998, phone interview by authors.

Chapter 10

1. The Associated Press, "World Bank recommends AIDS policy," (November 4, 1997), *Greensboro News & Record,* A-4.

2. Reuters, "Nigerian minister warns," October 21, 1997, America Online.

3. "Fighting the epidemic," (an interview with Michael Merson, MD, head of the World Health Organization's Global Program on AIDS), *Conference News,* (June 9, 1993), 2.

4. "AIDS: A global epidemic," *HIV & You,* (from the July 1996 International Conference on AIDS, Vancouver, British Columbia), http://www.hivpositive.com/f-HIVyou/f-Statistics/UN-AIDS.html, 7.

5. "Community care in developing countries," *Conference News*, (June 11, 1993), 6.

6. Bernice Powell Jackson, "Ethics and AIDS," *The Hartford Inquirer*, (Vol. 23, No. 21, October 22, 1997), 5.

7. *HIV/AIDS Ministries Network Focus Paper #21*, (New York: September 1993), Health and Welfare Program Ministries Department, General Board of Global Ministires, United Methodist Church, 3-9.

8. Stephen Brown, "Churches told to put aside differences on sexuality to fight AIDS," (September 26, 1996), Ecumenical News Service, www.igc.org/conferences/wfn.news/entries/756980628.html.

9. Bill Black, "HIV/AIDS and the church: Kenyan religious leaders become partners in prevention," *AIDScaptions*, (June 1997), 26.

10. *HIV/AIDS Ministries Network Focus Paper #21* (New York: September 1993), Health and Welfare Program Ministries Department, General Board of Global Ministries, United Methodist Church, 3.

Bibliography

"AIDS: A global epidemic." *HIV & You,* July 1996 International Conference on AIDS, Vancouver, BC, http://www.hivpositive.com/f-HIVyou/f-Statistics/ UNAIDS.html. 7.

"AIDS issue fades among Americans." *The Gallup Poll: Public Releases from Gallup Poll Results,* (1997), www.gallup.com/poll/news/97017.html.

American Association for World Health. "World AIDS day 1996. One world. One hope." (Washington, DC, 1996), 6-8.

"Americans worry over AIDS." *Reuters,* December 4, 1997, http://204.202.137. 113/sections/living/aidssurvey1204/index.html.

Amos, William E. *When AIDS Comes to Church.* Philadelphia, PA: Westminster Press, 1988.

Anderson, Gregory. "HIV prevention and older people." *Seicus Report* (December 1994/January 1995): 9-22.

"Apology paves way." *The Chronicle,* Winston-Salem, NC, May 22, 1997, 12.

Ashe, Arthur and Rampersad, Arnold. *Days of Grace.* Thorndike, ME: G.K. Hall and Co., 1993.

Balm in Gilead, Inc. "The African American clergy's declaration of war against AIDS." Resolution adopted at the First African American Religious Leaders Summit on HIV/AIDS, Washington, DC, February 28, 1995.

Bates, Karen Grigsley. "Black sexuality: The stereotypes have taken their toll." *Emerge* (April 1992) 45-48.

Black, Bill. "HIV/AIDS and the church: Kenyan religious leaders become partners in prevention," *AIDScaptions,* June 1997, 26.

"Black ministers say their churches should battle AIDS." *Baltimore Afro-American*, March 1, 1997: A-12.

Blendon, Robert J., Donelan, Karen, and Knox, Richard. "Public opinion and AIDS." In *AIDS, Ethics and Religion,* Kenneth R. Overberg (Ed.), 143-157. Maryknoll, NY: Orbis Books, 1944.

Boykin, Keith. *One More River to Cross: Black and Gay in America.* New York: Doubleday, 1996.

Briggs, Kenya. "A look at conflict and opportunities for dialogue between African American and lesbian/gay/bisexual communities." *Crossroads*, (February 1994), America Online.

Britton, Mariah. "Breaking the silence." *Yes! Journal of Positive Futures,* (Winter 1997-1998): 30-31.

Brown, Ronald E. and Reese Laura A. "The effects of religious messages on racial identity and systems blame among African Americans." *The Journal of Politics*, Volume 57 (1995): 24-43.

Carson, Emmett. *A Hand Up: Black Philanthropy and Self-Help in America.* Washington, DC: Joint Center for Political Studies, 1993.

Carten, Alma J. and Fennoy, Ilene. "African American families and HIV/AIDS: Caring for surviving children." *Child Welfare,* Vol.76 (1997): 107-125.

Carter, Nancy A. "Women don't get AIDS: They just die from it." *HIV/AIDS Ministries Network Focus Paper,* no. 17 (April 1992).

Chanoff, David and Elders, Joycelyn. *Joycelyn Elders M.D. From Sharecropper's Daughter to Surgeon General of the United States of America.* New York: William Morrow and Company, 1996.

"Churches against AIDS to hold prayer week." *Afro-American,* March 1, 1997: A-12.

"Community care in developing countries." *Conference News,* June 11, 1993, 6.

Cone, James E and Wilmore, Gayraud S. (Eds.). *Black Theology: A Documentary History; Volume II 1980-1992.* Maryknoll, NY: Orbis Books, 1993.

Cone, James H. *A Black Theology of Liberation: Twentieth Anniversary Edition.* Maryknoll, NY: Orbis Books, 1990.

Cooper, Mario. "The AIDS crisis within the African-American Community." *Themis.* Vol. 1, Issue 1, October/November 1997. http://www.iapac.org/minorities/themis.html), 6.

Corea, Gena. *The Invisible Epidemic: The Story of Women and AIDS.* New York: Harper Collins Publishers, 1992.

Countryman, L. William. *Dirt, Greed and Sex.* Philadelphia, PA: Fortress Press, 1988.

Dossey, Larry. *Healing Words: The of Prayer and the* Practice *of Medicine.* San Francisco, CA: Harper Collins Publishers, 1993.

Dyson, Michael E. *Race Rules.* New York: Addison-Wesley Publishing Company, 1996.

Felder, Cain Hope. *Troubling Biblical Waters: Race, Class, and Family.* Maryknoll, NY: Orbis Books, 1989.

"Fighting the epidemic." (Interview with Michael Merson, MD, head of WHO's Global Program on AIDS), *Conference News,* June 9, 1993, 2.

Fortunato, John. *AIDS: The Spiritual Dilemma.* San Francisco, CA: Harper and Row Publishers, 1987.

Gite, Lloyd. "The new agenda of the black church: Economic development for black America," *Black Enterprise,* December 1993: 54-59.

Gleghorn, A. A., Jemmott, J. B., Celentano, D.D., Kibourn, K.M. " Magic Johnson's HIV status: Impact on African-American STD patients." Paper presented at American Psychological Association, Toronto, Canada, August, 1993.

Graham, Rhonda. "And the choir sings on." *Wilmington News Journal,* October 23, 1994, America Online.

Greaser, Frances B. *And a Time to Die.* Scottdale, PA: Herald Press, 1995.

Greeley, Alexandra. "Concern about AIDS in minority communities," *FDA Consumer.* December 1995. http://www.fda.gov/fdac/features/095_aids.html.

Greeley, Andrew M. "Religion and attitudes toward AIDS policy." In *AIDS, Ethics and Religion: Embracing a World of Suffering,* Kenneth R. Overberg (Ed.), 223-230. Maryknoll, NY: Orbis Books, 1994.

Guess, Jerry M. "Freedom's warriors: The fighting black clergy, a historical view," *Crisis,* June/July, 1990, 30.

Hallaman, David G. (Ed.) *AIDS Issues: Confronting the Challenge.* New York: Pilgrim Press, 1989.

Harris, Forrest E. *Ministry for Social Crisis: Theology and Praxis in the Black Church Tradition.* Macon, GA: Mercer University Press, 1993.

Harris, James H. *Pastoral Theology: A Black Perspective.* Minneapolis, MN: Fortress Press, 1991.

Harry, Cheryl. "A black church's response to AIDS." Letter to the Editor in *Winston-Salem Chronicle,* December 12, 1996: A-8.

Harvard AIDS Institute. "Leading for life: The AIDS crisis among African Americans." A Report from the First Leading for Life Summit: Cambridge, MA. October 22, 1996.

Herek, Gregory and Capitanio, John. "Public reaction to AIDS in the United States: A second decade of stigma." *American Journal of Public Health,* Vol. 83, No. 4, April 1993, 576.

Herek, Gregory and Capitanio, John. "Black heterosexuals' attitudes toward lesbian and gay men in the United States." *The Journal of Sex Research,* Vol. 32, 1995, 95-105.

Herek, Gregory and Capitanio, John. "AIDS stigma and contact with persons with AIDS: Effects of direct and vicarious contact." *Journal of Applied Social Psychology,* Vol. 27, No. 1, 1997, 1-36.

Hunter, T. L., Kalichman, S. C., Russell, R. L., Sarwer, D. B., "Earwin 'Magic' Johnson's HIV serostatus disclosure: Effects of men's perceptions of AIDS." *Journal of Consulting and Clinical Psychology,* Vol. 61: 887-891.

International Conference on HIV in Children and Mothers. Published Press Release. Edinburgh, England: September 7, 1993. Referenced in *HIV/AIDS Ministries Network Focus Paper,* no.3 (February 17, 1989), America Online.

Jackson, Bernice P. "Ethics and AIDS," *The Hartford Inquirer,* Vol. 23, No. 21, October 22, 1997, 5.

Jackson, Edgar N. *The Many Faces of Grief.* Nashville, TN: Abingdon Press: 1988.

Kalichman, Seth C. "Magic Johnson and public attitudes toward AIDS: A review of empirical findings," *AIDS Education and Prevention,* Vol. 6, No. 6, 1994, 545.

Lawrence, Beverly H. *Reviving the Spirit.* New York: Grove Press, 1996.

Lewter, Nicholas Cooper and Mitchell Henry. *Soul Theology: The Heart of Black Culture.* Nashville, TN: Abington Press, 1991.

Lincoln, C. Eric. *The Black Experience in Religion.* Garden City, NY: Anchor/Doubleday, 1974.

Lincoln, C. Eric and Mamiya, Lawrence. *The Black Church in the African American Experience.* Durham, NC: Duke University Press, 1990.

Lyons, Cathy. "AIDS: A covenant to care." *HIV/AIDS Ministries Network Focus Paper,* no. 6 (1989), 1-8.

McCrary, Carolyn. "Interdependence as a normative value in pastoral counseling with African Americans." *The Journal of the I.T.C.,* Vol. XVIII, Nos. 1 and 2, Fall/Spring 1990/1991, 143.

Meckler, Laura. "AIDS compared to civil rights fight." (July 29, 1998), The Associated Press, 1-2.

Migliore, Daniel L. *Faith Seeking Understanding: An Introduction to Christian Theology.* Grand Rapids, MI: W.M.B. Eerdmans Publishing Company, 1991, 104-106.

Miller, Kenneth. "A Church for the Twenty-First Century." *Life,* April, 1997, 50.

Nations, Don, "10 assurances of pastoral care for those infected or affected by HIV/AIDS," *HIV/AIDS Ministries Network Focus Paper #22,* November, 1993. Health and Welfare Program Ministries Program Department, General Board of Global Ministries, The United Methodist Church, 5.

Mitchell, Angela. "Risky sex: Risky candid talk about responsible behavior." *Emerge,* (March 1992), 26-32.

Moore, David W. "AIDS issue fades among Americans." *The Gallup Poll,* http//www.gallup.com/poll/news/971017.html.

Morrissey, Paul F. *Let Someone Hold You: The Journey of a Hospice Priest.* New York: Crossroad, 1994.

Morrissey, Paul F. "In Bronx, amid death, people still hope." *National Catholic Reporter,* (September 15, 1995), America Online.

Muhammad, Abdul A. "HIV/AIDS in the African-American community." Nation of Islam Ministry of Health and Human Services, (July 29, 1997), http://www.noihealth.org/hivedu.html, 1.

The Names Project Foundation. "Guidelines for the interfaith quilt project." San Francisco, CA: November 2, 1994.

Nations, Don. "Guidelines for the giving of pastoral care to those persons who are infected/affected by HIV/AIDS." *HIV/AIDS Ministries Network Focus Paper, No. 22* (November 1993): 3-4.

Nations, Don. "10 assurances of pastoral care for those infected or affected by HIV/AIDS." *HIV/AIDS Ministries Network Focus Paper, No. 22,* New York (November 1993), 5. Health and Welfare Program Ministries Program Department, General Board of Global Ministries, United Methodist Church.

New Oxford Annotated Bible, The (New Revised Standard Edition). New York, NY: Oxford University Press, 1991.

Norris, Mackie H. "The black church and the AIDS crisis." *HIV/AIDS Ministries Network Focus Paper, no. 29* (December 1995): 1-10.

Nungesser, L.G. *Epidemic of Courage: Facing AIDS in America.* New York: St. Martin's Press, 1986.

Perelli, Robert J. *Ministry to Persons with AIDS: A Family Systems Approach.* Minneapolis, MN: Augsburg Press, 1991.

Rimer, Sara. "Blacks urged to increase awareness of AIDS epidemic," *The New York Times News service,* October 23, 1996, 1-2, http://plato.divanet.com/mansco/qnn/1996/hv6oct/HV207003.TXT.

Rosin, Hanna. "The homecoming," (June 5, 1995), *The New Republic,* 22.

Rotello, Gabriel. "Watch out: Al Sharpton ACTS UP." *New York Newsday,* January 6, 1994, America Online.

Russell, Letty M. (Ed.). *The Church with AIDS.* Louisville, KY: Westminster/John Knox Press, 1990.

Sawyer, Mary R. *Black Ecumenism: Implementing the Demands of Justice.* Valley Forge, PA: Trinity Press, International, 1994.

Shelp, Earle E. *AIDS and the Church in the Second Decade.* Philadelphia, PA: Westminster/John Knox Press, 1992.

Shelp, Earle E. and Sunderland, Ronald. *AIDS and the Church.* Philadelphia, PA: Westminster Press, 1988.

Smith, Walter J. *AIDS Living and Dying with Hope: Issues in Pastoral Care.* New York: Paulist Press, 1988.

Stevenson, Howard C. "The psychology of sexual racism and AIDS: An ongoing saga of distrust and the sexual other." *Journal of Black Studies,* volume 25 (1994): 62-81.

Stewart, Carlyle F. *African-American Church Growth: 12 Principles for Prophetic Ministry.* Nashville, TN: Abington Press, 1994.

Stirton, Timothy. "Man with a mission." *The Crisis,* Vol. 98, No. 6 (June/July 1990): 48-50.

Straub, Debra G., ed., "Joycelyn Elders." In *Voices of Multicultural America.* Detroit: Gale Research, 1996, 359.

Stryker, Jeff. "Tuskegee's long arm still touches a nerve." (April 13, 1997). *The New York Times,* http://www.drugfreeamerica.org/inhale_ne.html, 1-3.

Tapia, Andres. "Soul searching: How is the black church responding to the urban crisis?" *Christianity Today,* (March 1996), reprinted in Harambee Archives, http://www.harambee.org/archive/soul.html, 9.

Thomas, Robert. "Heaven's bleach will your AIDS virus." *Nashville Pride,* (October 18, 1997): 4.

Tillman, Otis, MD. *A Prescription for the Soul: Prayers and Meditations.* High Point, NC: The Marshall Group, 1995.

The United Methodist Church. *The Book of Resolutions of the United Methodist Church.* Nashville, TN: United Methodist Publishing House, 1996.

United Methodist News Service. "Eight agencies addressing HIV/AIDS receive grants from mission board." Published Press Release (January 6, 1997), America Online.

U.S. Department of Health and Human Services, Centers for Disease Control and Prevention. "Morbidity and mortality weekly report." Atlanta, GA: CDC, September 9, 1994.

U.S. Department of Health and Human Services, Centers for Disease Control and Prevention. "CDC fact sheet—Facts about women and AIDS." Atlanta, GA: CDC, February 3, 1995.

U.S. Department of Health and Human Services, Centers for Disease Control and Prevention. "Morbidity and mortality weekly report." Atlanta, GA: CDC, February 3, 1995.

U.S. Department of Health and Human Services, Centers for Disease Control and Prevention. "Current trends I: Update, acquired immunodeficiency syndrome—United States, 1995." Atlanta, GA: CDC, 1996.

U.S. Department of Health and Human Services, National Institute of Health. "Older americans at risk of HIV take few precautions." Bethesda, MD: CDC, January 4, 1994.

Walker, Theodore Jr. *Empower the People: Social Ethics for the African- American Church.* Maryknoll, NY: Orbis Books, 1991.

Washington, Harriet. "HIV Among African Americans." *Harvard AIDS Review,* Spring/Summer 1996, http://www.hsph.harvard.edu/Organizations/hai_ini/publicat/review/sprsum_96.html, 6.

White, Evelyn. "Identity crisis for the black church." *San Francisco Chronicle,* January 12, 1994, America Online.

Whitfield, Leroy. "Black Plague." *Positively Aware,* (September/October 1997), Vol. 8, No. 5, 46.

Williams, Cecil with Lard, Rebecca. *No Hiding Place: Empowerment and Recovery for Our Troubled Communities.* San Francisco, CA: Harper Collins Publishers, 1992.

Wimberly, Edward P. *African American Pastoral Care.* Nashville, TN: Abington Press, 1991.

Wimberly, Edward P. "Pastoral counseling with African-American males." *The Journal of the I.T.C.,* Vol. XXI, Nos. 1 and 2, Fall/Spring 1993/1994, 127-144.

Woodward, James (Ed.). *Embracing the Chaos: Theological Responses to AIDS.* London: SPCK, 1990.

"World Bank recommends AIDS policy." *Greensboro News & Record,* November 4, 1997, A-4.

Index

"I know how you feel," avoiding
    saying, 66
Immunex, 75
Incarceration, and AIDS risk, 15
Insurance, and AIDS, 15
International Association of
    Physicians in AIDS Care, 7
International HIV/AIDS Conference
    (Berlin, Germany), 95
Intervention, AIDS, 102-104
"Is Theology Possible After AIDS?,"
    35

Jackson, Bernice Powell, *xi-xiii*,94
Jesus, and gays, 23
Johnson, Earvin "Magic," 26
Johnson, Sam, 79
Jokomo, Christopher, 92
Jones, Cleve, 88
Juvenile AIDS victims, 27

Kaiser Family Foundation, 27-28
Kalichman, S. C., 26
Kanyoro, Musimbi, 96
Kauma (Bishop), 98
Kaunda, Kenneth, 92
Kemron, 75
Kenyan Christian AIDS Network, 97
Kilbourn, K. M., 26
King-McCoy, Ernestine, 76

Lartey, Seth, 46,83-84
Leading for Life Summit, 7
Liberation theology, 3-4,37
Lincoln, C. Eric, 1,2,10,36,60
Long haul, 66-67

Mamiya, Lawrence H., 1,2,60
Mann, Jonathan, 94
MAP Kenya HIV/AIDS Project,
    96-97

Matthews, Charles, 16
McCrary, Carolyn, 62
McCray, George, 47,79,85
McKinney, George, 6
Ministers, at funerals of AIDS
    victims, 19
Minority AIDS Project, 75-76
MOVERS (Minorities Overcoming
    the Virus through Education,
    Responsibility, and
    Spirituality), 79
Mt. Tabor Missionary Baptist
    Church, 79-80
Muhammed, Abdul Alim, 16,73
"My Body, God's Temple," 57

NAACP, 3
The Names Project Foundation,
    88-89
Nation of Islam (NOI) Ministry
    of Health and Human
    Services, 73-75
National African-American Church
    AIDS Council, 73
National Anti-Drug Campaign,
    70-71
National Baptist Convention, U.S.A.
    (NBCUSA), 24
National Black Religious Summit
    on Sexuality (1997), 7
    consensus statement, 42-43
National Institute of Healthcare
    Research, 47
National Institutes of Health, 94
National Interfaith Quilt Program, 89
National Science Foundation, 27
National Urban League, 3
Nations, Don, 61
Ninth International Congress
    on HIV/AIDS, 98
No Hiding Place, 35,38,59

One More River to Cross, 27